NEUROLOGY – LABORATORY AND CLINICAL RESEARCH DEVELOPMENTS

BODY IN MIND

A NEW LOOK AT THE SOMATOSENSORY CORTICES

NEUROLOGY – LABORATORY AND CLINICAL RESEARCH DEVELOPMENTS

Cerebral Ischemia
R.H. Rosenwasser (Editor)
ISBN: 1-56072-137-5

Intracranial Hypertension
Stefan Mircea Iencean and Alexandru Vladimir Ciurea
2009. ISBN: 978-1-60741-862-7
2009. ISBN: 978-1-60876-549-2 (E-book)

Cerebral Blood Flow Regulation
Nodar P. Mitagvaria and Haim (James) I. Bicher
2009. ISBN: 978-1-60692-163-0
2009. ISBN: 978-1-60741-405-6 (E-book)

Cerebral Ischemia in Young Adults: Pathogenic and Clinical Perspectives
Alessandro Pezzini and Alessandro Padovani (Editors)
2009. ISBN: 978-1-60741-627-2

Dizziness: Vertigo, Disequilibrium and Lightheadedness
Agnes Lindqvist and Gjord Nyman (Editors)
2009. ISBN: 978-1-60741-847-4
2009. ISBN: 978-1-61668-001-5 (E-book)

Somatosensory Cortex: Roles, Interventions and Traumas
Niels Johnsen and Rolf Agerskov (Editors)
2009. ISBN: 978-1-60741-876-4

Cognitive Impairment: Causes, Diagnosis and Treatment
Melanie L. Landow (Editor)
2009. ISBN: 978-1-60876-205-7

Dystonia: Causes, Symptoms and Treatment
Josué Kurstot and Maurice Forsström (Editors)
2009. ISBN: 978-1-60876-445-7

Handbook of Spinal Cord Injuries: Types, Treatments and Prognosis
Tanya C. Berkovsky (Editor)
2010. ISBN: 978-1-60876-002-2

Women and Multiple Sclerosis
Duane O'Mahony and Anrai de Búrca (Editors)
2009. ISBN: 978-1-60876-070-1

Neurological Lists
Mohammad Zare, Farzad Fatehi, Mohammad Saadatnia and Keivan Basiri
2010. ISBN: 978-1-60876-351-1

Body in Mind: A New Look at the Somatosensory Cortices
Michael Schaefer
2010. ISBN: 978-1-60876-955-1

NEUROLOGY – LABORATORY AND CLINICAL RESEARCH DEVELOPMENTS

BODY IN MIND

A NEW LOOK AT THE SOMATOSENSORY CORTICES

MICHAEL SCHAEFER

Nova Science Publishers, Inc.
New York

For permission to use material from this book please contact us:
Telephone 631-231-7269; Fax 631-231-8175
Web Site: http://www.novapublishers.com

LIBRARY OF CONGRESS CATALOGING-IN-PUBLICATION DATA

Schaefer, Michael, 1952-
Body in mind : a new look at the somatosensory cortices / Michael Schaefer.
p. ; cm.
Includes bibliographical references and index.
ISBN 978-1-60876-955-1 (softcover)
1. Sensorimotor cortex. 2. Somesthesia. I. Title.
[DNLM: 1. Somatosensory Cortex--physiology. 2. Body Image. 3. Neuronal Plasticity--physiology. 4. Phantom Limb--rehabilitation. 5. Social Perception. WL 307 S294b 2009]
QP383.15.S33 2009
612.8'11--dc22

2009050561ISBN: 978-1-60876-955-1

Published by Nova Science Publishers, Inc. ✢ New York

CONTENTS

Preface		**vii**
Chapter 1	Introduction: Jeff's Hand	**1**
Chapter 2	Long-Term Plasticity in SI: Phantom Limbs and the Existence of the Soul	**5**
Chapter 3	Short-Term Modulations in SI: How Using a Tool Can Change Body Image and Other Examples of Top-Down Mechanisms in SI	**11**
Chapter 4	SI Represents the Perceived Rather than the Physical Image of the Body	**23**
Chapter 5	The Twofold Character of Touch: Viewing the Body Magnified	**27**
Chapter 6	Morphing the Body	**35**
Chapter 7	My Body and Your Body: SI and the Social World	**45**
Chapter 8	Dr. Strangelove and the Evil Hand	**55**
Chapter 9	Using the Dynamic Facet of the Body Image for Neurorehabilitation	**61**
Chapter 10	Conclusion: Consequences for the Image of Our Self	**65**
References		**71**
Index		**81**

PREFACE

How do we perceive our bodies and where are they represented in our brains? For decades, it has been known that the primary somatosensory cortex (or SI), located on the postcentral gyrus, codes the surface of our bodies in a topographical way. Classic studies understand this body map representation in SI as fixed and reflecting the physical location of peripheral stimulation in the form of the famous somatosensory homunculus. This book reports results of recent studies that challenge this view and suggest a more complex role of SI. Animal studies provided first evidence to this new understanding of SI. These experiments employed simple tactile illusions to show that SI reflects the perceived rather than the physical location of peripheral stimulation. Using similar illusions (in particular by manipulating visuo-tactile integration processes), studies with human subjects confirmed those findings. Moreover, recent studies demonstrated that we do not necessarily have to evoke a tactile illusion to affect the perception of the body and its representation in SI. Even a simple "disguising" of the body seems to be sufficient to affect the perception of the body, along with corresponding changes in the topography of SI! This shows that the topographic representation in SI may adapt extremely dynamically to different situational requirements. Furthermore, there is exciting new evidence that SI responds differentially when observed touch is attributed to the own body compared to another body—in both cases in absence of any real touch! This has led to the conclusion that the somatosensory cortices may even be involved in processes of social perception. The new insights about the functions of SI may contribute to our understanding of body perception and also encourage approaches focusing on dynamic aspects of the body image for future therapeutic interventions. But the consequences might be even more fundamental. Touch is always twofold. It bears information about an external object touching the skin and at the same time about the body itself. Thus, the investigation of the perception of the body also has an impact on the image of the self. This book also tries to discuss the outcome of research on body perception in the light of the meaning for the understanding of the self.

Chapter 1

INTRODUCTION: JEFF'S HAND

Just a hand? Is it part of a new advertising campaign? If so, what for? The citizens of the capital of the USA probably were wondering what these huge images of a hand were about. From July 2003 through January 2004, people in Washington, D.C., viewed billboards in different places in the city depicting always the same image—simply the palm of an open hand. These temporary billboard installations were part of an art project directed by the Cuban-born artist Felix Gonzales-Torres at the Smithsonian's Hirshhorn Museum. The reproduction of this single image in multiple citywide locations was caused by the intention of the artist to make art more accessible to a wider public. Gonzales-Torres (1957-1996) named the work *Untitled (For Jeff)*. The title of the work points to the name of a healthcare worker who nursed the artist's dying friend. Seeing the open hand in various contexts probably led to a range of possible associations, depending on the location and environment in which each billboard was sited. The hand may have symbolized assistance, offered welcome, or searched for support. It may also remind the audience of the transience of all beings.

The relationship between body and mind has always been an important question, not only for artists. It is a classic philosophical problem. For many philosophers such as, for instance, the French phenomenologist Maurice Merlau-Ponty, this relationship was a core issue of our being in the world (see his *Phenomenology of Perception,* 1945). One description of this problem is that on one hand, I *have* a body, but on the other hand I *am* also my body.

So how shall we treat our body? Is it our "friend?" Or "foe?" Or, is it just some flesh we have that should not be allowed to get to dominant over our mind? And what is the body? Everything below the head? Or does the body include our head and brain? Or perhaps parts of our brain, which apparently do not have anything to do with cognitive thinking, e.g., the parietal and occipital lobes? Does, regarding people who suffer from depression, the statement really make sense that they *themselves* are not sick: It's only my brain that has problems with some neurotransmitters, but not me—me, myself, I am ok. This is the way one of the main characters of Jonathan Franzen's great novel *The Corrections* has described it (Franzen et al., 2001).

Although we do not have a clear answer how to regard and manage the relation to the body and what, for example, the exact borders are, as healthy adults, we are used to the presence and shape of the body, and usually we do not spend much time on reasoning about this strange question. But it was not always like that. If we observe babies, who are just a couple of months old, we sometimes can see how they just discover that the small hands, which used to move in front of their faces, belong to themselves, that these hands are their own hands, following their commands and being a part of their identity. This discovery is so fascinating for them that they luckily look again and again at their hands, moving them a little bit and spending much time on this intriguing new thing.

Only recently, the role of the body and its representation in the brain became an exciting new research topic in the field of neurosciences. The ownership and embodiment of one's body is essential for successful interaction with the environment. At first glance, the ownership of one's body seems to be trivial. However, recent studies have demonstrated that bodily experience can be manipulated in a very fast and easy way, resulting in disturbances of feelings—what belongs to the body and what not. For example, only few experimental manipulations are necessary to incorporate artificial limbs in body image (Botvinick and Cohen, 1998). Moreover, similar manipulations can put us "out" of the body and into an alien body (Lenggenhager et al., 2007). The current book reviews recent studies on body representations and perceptual aspects of the bodily-self including illusory manipulations of self-attribution and embodiment. Thereby, it focuses on the role for the primary somatosensory cortex (SI) for the perception of the body. The book suggests a model where SI maintains an important early image of the body that is crucial for perceptual aspects of the body as well as for disturbances of this perception during illusory manipulations, operating both via automatic bottom-up and also top-down processes. Thus, a more complex role for SI, the first cortical site contributing to the processing of tactile information, is proposed. The core thesis will be that SI seems to code the *perceived* image of the body rather than solely representing physical information on the body surface.

The sense of touch carries information about an external object touching the skin and at the same time about the body itself. Based on this dual nature of touch

(Serino and Haggard, 2009), recent studies even suggest that this early concept of our own body may also include important dimensions of our self. Thus, the tactile sense and its first major processing area in SI seem to be essential for building a first representation of our body and self. This is also supported by expressions like "let's keep in touch," or to feel "touched" by someone's behavior.

Below, I will trace how studies based on neuroimaging data have contributed to this new view on SI. I will first review studies that focused on changes in the functional topography of SI after amputation of a limb. These long-term plastic changes in SI have been reported both in humans with phantom-limb pain as well as in animals after deafferentation. In a second step, I will focus on changes in SI that occur much more rapidly. These short-term modulations have been linked to specific tasks and also to tool use, suggesting influences of areas in the frontal lobe on somatosensory processing. The next chapter will discuss the central hypothesis of this book, suggesting that the topographic map in SI represents the perceived rather than the "physical" image of the body. The following two chapters will concentrate on perceptual illusions and morphed bodies, thereby trying to provide support for the outlined hypothesis. The next chapters will review the role of SI for social aspects of behavior. The subsequent chapter will introduce patient W.H., who was diagnosed to have the alien hand syndrome. I will use this exciting case study to ask for the organization of body perception in this bizarre movement disorder. In the following chapter, I then will discuss the question if and how recent research may help people who have impaired somatosensory abilities (a frequent consequence, for example, after stroke). Finally, I will try to think about possible impacts of the results of these studies on the image of our self, perhaps helping us to understand why a simple image of the palm of a hand can be so meaningful for us.

Chapter 2

Long-Term Plasticity in SI: Phantom Limbs and the Existence of the Soul

Every year, many Europeans spend their holidays on the beautiful island Tenerife, which belongs to Spain but is located close to the West African coast. While having a great time on this volcano island, they may also encounter a famous canon named "El tigre," which is placed at the entrance of the harbour of the island. The story of the "El tigre" goes back to the end of the 18th century. Since he was getting an upgrade to be now a "Rear Admiral of the Blue," the year 1797 was starting really successful for the famous British admiral Lord Nelson. However, at the end of this year, he lost his fortune. For years, the English marine struggled with the Spanish marine for ruling the Canary Islands, where the island of Tenerife was the most important one. Nelson tried to capture a Spanish ship at Santa Cruz de Tenerife. It must have been a terrible battle for Lord Nelson. Suddenly, he was wounded at the elbow. Unfortunately the injury was very deep, which made an amputation of the whole right arm up to the shoulder necessary. But soon after the amputation, Admiral Lord Nelson experienced astonishing feelings: He strongly felt compelling phantom-limb pain, including the sensation of fingers digging into his phantom palm. These strange ghostly feelings led him to proclaim that this phantom was a "direct proof of the existence of the soul." Since parts of the body can survive physical destruction, the entire person may also survive the death of the body (Riddoch, 1941; Ramachandran and Hirstein, 1998).

The term phantom limb was first used by Silas Weir Mitchell (1871, 1872), followed by many case reports of phantom-limb feelings. The experience of phantom limbs was so astonishing that it fascinated an audience far beyond scientists and physicians. Often, these reports were regarded as clinical curiosities rather than being subjects of experimental studies. This is why the first description of this case by Silas W. Mitchell was published in a popular magazine instead of a medical or scientific journal. Even today, we are still fascinated when we hear patients reporting phantom-limb phenomena. Perhaps this can also be explained by the way pictures of amputees have been melted with the literary genre of sea heroes in the 18th and 19th centuries, with the most prominent figure of Captain Ahab, main character of the great American novel *Moby Dick* by Herman Melville. Besides being stuff for literature, the emergence of phantom-limb pain also fascinated philosophers. For example, Maurice Merleau-Ponty used these phenomena for thoughts on how our perception in general may work (Merleau-Ponty, 1945).

With the emergence of new neuroimaging techniques, the examination of these phenomena has been getting again into the focus of scientists. As we can see below, recent studies on phantom limbs provided important insights for neural plasticity in the adult brain.

In 1937, Penfield and Boldrey were the first ones who discovered that a region on the human postcentral gyrus represents the surface of the body in a topographic map: the primary somatosensory cortex or SI (Figure 1). Any physical stimulation of the body surface is represented in this primary somatosensory area. Moreover, this map shows systematically the tactile sensitivity of each body area. Body parts with low receptor densities (e.g., the back) are represented by small areas in SI, and body parts with a high sensitivity to tactile stimulation (e.g., the tongue) are represented by relatively big areas. Thus, the resulting body image in SI is distorted in the form of the famous somatosensory homunculus.

For decades, researchers believed that the topography in SI is fixed already in early childhood. More in general, it has been believed that no new neural connections can be formed in the adult mammalian brain: once those connections were built in early life, it was assumed that they would remain fixed for the whole life. This was also used as an explanation why people learn very fast in childhood but rather slowly when they are adults. Similarly, this theory has also been used to explain why there is often so little functional recovery after damage to the nervous system.

This traditional view of an unchangeable body map representation in SI was questioned by animal studies conducted by Merzenich and colleagues (1984). Several experiments revealed that the amputation of a finger yielded in plastic changes in SI. For example, two months after amputation of the middle finger of adult monkeys, they found that the area of cortex corresponding to this digit was responding to tactile stimuli delivered to the adjacent digits. Thus, this area has been "taken over" by tactile input of the adjacent fingers.

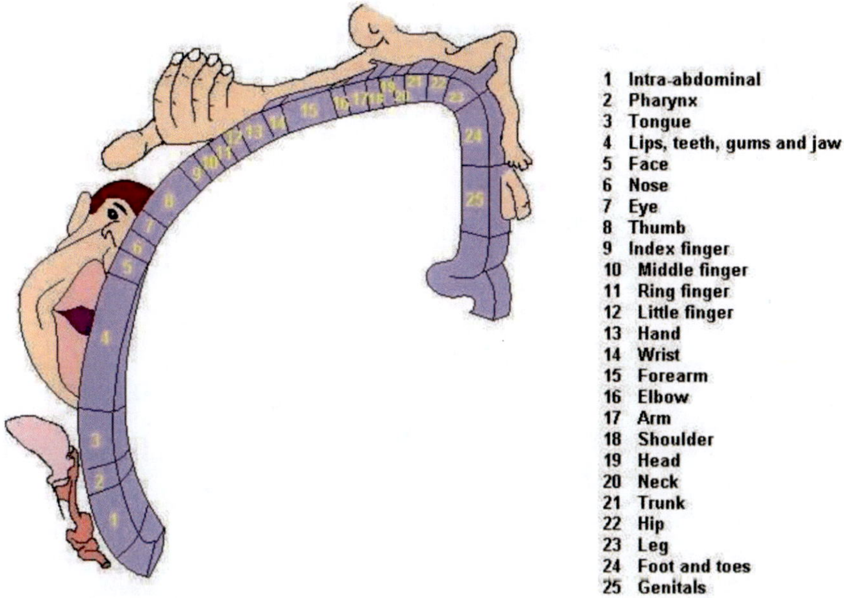

Figure 1. The primary somatosensory cortex on the postcentral gyrus and the parts of the body it is concerned with (cross-section through the cortex).

Similar experiments with monkeys were done by Pons et al. (1991). After deafferentation of an upper limb, they reported the cortical area once corresponding to the hand was taken over by sensory input from the face. But while the plastic changes in the studies by Merzenich et al. were about one millimeter, here, the results demonstrated sensory reorganization over a centimeter!

These results from animal data led to a new interest in studies with upper limb amputees. Amputees who have lost an extremity often vividly feel their phantom limb. Phantom-limb pain is a frequent consequence of the amputation of a body part occurring in up to 80% of all amputees (Jensen et al., 1983; Wartan et al., 1997). For example, a British study with war veterans who have lost a limb reported that 55% of them felt phantom-limb pain (Wartan et al., 1997). Some upper limb amputees also report referred sensations (Ramachandran, 1998; Ramachandran and Hirstein, 1998), meaning that they experience their phantom limb when stimulating specific intact parts of the body, which is then referred to the phantom limb.

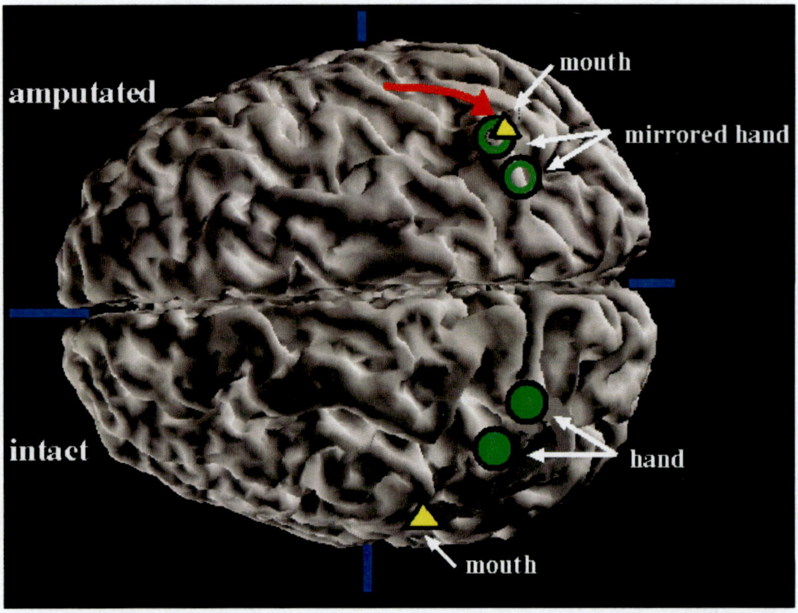

Figure 2. Cortical reorganization in upper limb amputees. The cortical representation of the mouth region (yellow triangle on the amputated side) was found to invade the region that formerly represented the amputated limb (see red arrow). This cortical shift of the mouth representation correlated highly with the magnitude of phantom-limb pain.

It has been discussed that these phantom-limb phenomena might result from distortions in the body map topography in SI (Ramachandran, 1998; Ramachandran and Hirstein, 1998). Since upper limb amputees have lost an arm and a hand, there is "empty space" in the functional topography in SI. No sensory information is coming to the region that has been formerly innervated by the hand and arm. Thus, many researchers speculated that the distorted body image might be responsible for phantom-limb phenomena (Ramachandran, 1998; Ramachandran and Hirstein, 1998). In 1994, Yang et al. employed the new technique of magnetoencephalography (MEG) and used neuromagnetic source imaging to map the topography in SI in upper limb amputees. They found that the cortical representation of the mouth region invaded the region that formerly represented the amputated limb (see Figure 2). This cortical reorganization was a prominent example of plastic changes in the brain. Thus, even the adult brain seems to be able to change after injuries. Subsequent research extended these reports by showing that these plastic changes are not related to all phantom-limb phenomena, but are strongly correlated with the degree of phantom-limb pain (Flor et al., 1995).

While these results point to a maladaptive plasticity in SI, there are also examples for a beneficial plasticity. By using neuromagnetic source imaging, Elbert et al. (1995) demonstrated that the cortical representation of the digits of the left hand of string players was larger than that of a control group. Moreover, the amount of cortical reorganization in the representation of the finger digits was correlated with the age at which the person started to play strings. The authors concluded that the topographic organization in SI depends on use, and it adapts to current needs and experiences of the individual.

Thus, there seems to a "bad" plastic reorganization in the case of phantom-limb pain as well "good" or beneficial plastic changes as a result of behavioral-relevant training or learning. In a study conducted by Flor et al. (2001), the idea was to combine both mechanisms to help patients with phantom-limb pain. Thus, Flor et al. (2001) employed a sensory discrimination training to reverse both cortical reorganization and the associated phantom-limb pain. Five patients with arm amputations who underwent the training were compared to five patients who received standard medical treatment (including analgesic medication, transcutaneous nerve stimulation, or physical therapy). The patients participated in ten daily training sessions over duration of two weeks of a feedback-guided sensory training. In this training, they had to discriminate the frequency or location of high intensity non-painful electric stimuli applied through eight electrodes, which were attached to the stump in a region covering the median nerve. The results showed a significant improvement in the discrimination abilities of the patients. Cortical reorganization was measured by neuroelectric source imaging (using electroencephalography, EEG). The data revealed that the reorganization was reduced in the training but not in the control group. Moreover, the amount of the reduced cortical reorganization was positively associated with the improvement in sensory discrimination ability and also with the reduction of phantom-limb pain.

However, given the limited number of patients, this trial was mainly experimental. Nevertheless, the results are encouraging and suggest that the alteration of cortical reorganization by behavioral means might be an effective treatment for phantom-limb pain. As we will see later, other interventions based on manipulations of visual-tactile integration also seem to very promising. Thus, future therapeutic approaches may provide new ways in helping amputees with phantom-limb pain, a pain that in the past often was seen as untreatable for many patients.

Chapter 3

SHORT-TERM MODULATIONS IN SI: HOW USING A TOOL CAN CHANGE BODY IMAGE AND OTHER EXAMPLES OF TOP-DOWN MECHANISMS IN SI

Have you ever had an accident with your car? Perhaps you may remember that bumping with your car against a wall or another car may not only have damaged the car but also that you almost felt the touch as if it were on your own body. Even when a car only slightly touches something, we often have the impression to *feel* this touch, as if we had incorporated the shape of the car into our own body image. We are in a similar situation whenever we use a tool. For example, after working for hours with a screwdriver, we sometimes have the sensation to "feel" with the tip of this tool. In the same sense we often "feel" with the bumpers of the car when we try to park the car or when having an accident.

By demonstrating neural correlates for tool use, recent animal studies have shown that these examples are not only metaphors. When an external object is used as a tool, for example a screwdriver, it is felt as becoming a part or an extension of the arm. Thus, the tool has been incorporated into body image. In an intriguing study, Iriki et al. (1996) demonstrated the basis of this perceptual assimilation of tool and hand. Monkeys were trained to receive some food pellets by using a tong. Iriki et al. (1996) then used single cell recordings of neurons in the parietal cortex to find neurons that were associated with this tool use task. The authors were able to identify bimodal neurons in the anterior bank of the intraparietal sulcus (IPS) that were sensitive both for tactile and visual events and which appeared to code the schema of the hand. The fascinating result of this study was that Iriki et al. (1996) could demonstrate that during tool use the visual receptive fields of those cells changed dynamically. Thus, the receptive fields of these bimodal cells seemed to include the entire length of the tong or to cover the expanded accessible space, as if the hand was elongated to the tip of the tool. Hence, when we use a tool like a tong or a screwdriver, it seems that the body image adopts to incorporate this tool into the schema of the hand.

Using brain imaging methods, Obayashi et al. (2001) and Inoue et al. (2001) provided further support for this dynamic aspect of body image. Obayashi et al. (2001) explored brain areas in awake macaque monkeys during tool use by employing a positron emission tomography (PET) approach. They found tool use related increased activity in the intraparietal region, the basal ganglia, pre-supplementary motor area, premotor cortex, and the cerebellum, indicating a dynamic reorganization of reaching-related representations. In a similar study, Inoue et al. (2001) investigated normal human subjects performing a tool-use task also by using PET. They showed that in the right hand condition, the only site activated during tool use in comparison to a control condition (performing the task with fingers) was the lateral edge of the right IPS. In contrast, for the left hand condition, it was the middle part of the left IPS. Activation in the contralateral hemisphere failed to show significant results, suggesting a role of the ipsilateral posterior parietal cortex for visuosomatosensory integration when subjects use a tool.

The above-mentioned studies suggest that the ipsilateral posterior parietal cortex is crucial for integrating a tool into the body schema. Since tool use has to integrate visuo-tactile information, it is reasonable to associate it with the posterior parietal cortex (PPC), which is known to be related to multisensory integration. However, in the previous chapter, we have seen that phantom sensations as disturbances of the body schema also seem to be related to alterations in the somatosensory cortices. Phantom sensations sometimes occur as referred sensations (Ramachandran, 1998). Thus, for example, when the cheek of the patient is touched, he feels the thumb of this lost hand. These referred sensations are stable over time and occur in a topographic manner. Hence, when the patient's chin is being touched, he feels his pinky, when the upper lip is stimulated, he has the feeling to be touched on his index finger. Typically, other regions on the body also show these referred sensations, e.g., the back. However, in general, only few upper limb amputees report to have these referred sensations (Flor et al., 1995). While phantom-limb pain seems to be associated with the magnitude of the cortical reorganization in SI, the neural correlates of referred sensations remain unclear. Although some studies suggest involvement of primary and secondary somatosensory cortices (SII) and also PPC (Flor et al. 2000), further studies are necessary to clarify the neural mechanisms underlying these phenomena.

Phantom sensations can be compared to using a tool because in both cases occurs a referral of the sensation of the touch. When we use a tool, the sensory signals were referred off the body to the tip of a tool (Yamamoto and Kitazawa, 2001). Thus, it seems reasonable to hypothesize that the brain may represent the modified body schema during tool use through the activity of a distributed neural network including SI and SII. In order to test this hypothesis, we conducted an experiment where we asked subjects to manipulate a small object with a pair of tongs (as a tool) or with their hands (control condition) while recording their brain activity with MEG.

The aim of this study was to examine task-related changes in the somatosensory homunculus during tool use. Neuromagnetic source imaging seems to be a promising technique to detect even small alterations in the somatosensory homunculus. Methodological studies have revealed that this approach allows valid and reliable mapping of SI (e.g., Schaefer et al., 2002a,b; 2004a). We examined the functional topography of SI with a pneumatical tactile stimulation device while subjects were performing the tasks. The stimulation device consisted of a diaphragm with a 10-mm diameter, causing a distinct tactile sensation when inflated toward the skin by a pulse of pressed air of 2.5 atm for 20 ms (Figure 3). As stimulation devices were only a few millimeters in height, they were easily taped to the first (D1) and fifth digit (D5) in such a way that the participants were able to use the tongs with almost no restrictions. The participants were seated on a comfortable chair with their heads placed in the mould of the Dewar of a whole-head MEG system in a magnetically shielded room.

The experiment was organized in three blocks (tool condition, hand condition, rest condition). During each block, D1 and D5 were stimulated, resulting in 400 stimuli for each finger. Each block lasted for approximately ten minutes. In each of the blocks, the subjects were stimulated on D1 and D5 and told to ignore the tactile stimuli, not to move their heads and to concentrate on the task.

The task was analogue to that of the study by Inoue et al. (2001), but slightly changed due to the restrictions in the MEG environment. The participants were instructed to pick up a rubber cylinder from one target area and transfer it to the next target area. The target area was cued by beep sounds. In the hand condition, the subjects should transfer the cylinder with the thumbs and index fingers of their right hands. During the tool condition, the subjects had to perform the same task by using a pair of tongs. Thus, in both conditions, the participants performed the same task. In a third condition, the subjects had no task and were told to relax without making hand or other movements (rest condition).

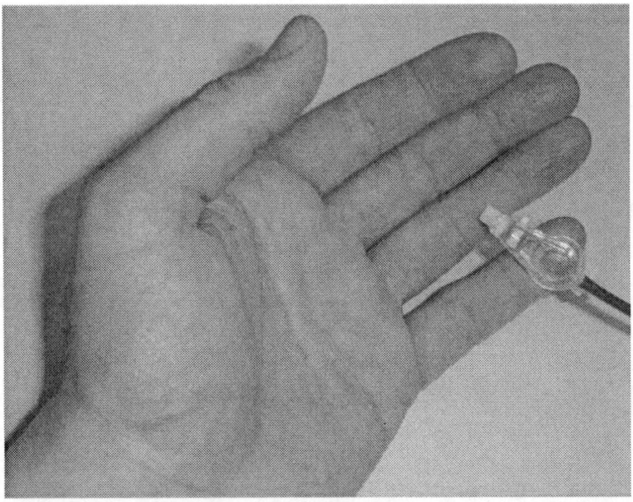

Figure 3. Picture of the pneumatically driven stimulation device. The device consisted of a diaphragm with a 10-mm diameter, causing a distinct tactile sensation when inflated toward the skin by a pulse of pressed air.

The behavioral performance was video controlled. Somatosensory evoked magnetic fields (SEFs) were recorded using a whole head MEG-system with 148 sensors. Somatotopic representations of the stimulated fingers were determined by source modeling of the earliest prominent activity peak of the magnetic brain response ranging in a time window from 35 to 85s (M60 component) (Elbert et al., 1995; Braun et al., 2001; Schaefer et al., 2006). The generator of the M60 component has been related to neural sources in cortical area 3b of SI by previous work (e.g., Hari et al., 1993). Ipsilateral activity was modeled by an additional source when it improved the explained variance (Zhu et al., 2007). To determine the neuromagnetic sources, dipole localizations were overlaid onto individual magnetic resonance images.

Changes in the topographical localization of D1 and D5 were then assessed using a distance measure between the equivalent dipole locations of D1 and D5. The dipole locations were specified in polar coordinates (Braun et al., 2001; Schaefer et al., 2006). Cortical shifts along the postcentral gyrus were expressed by polar angle $\Delta\vartheta$, which describes shifts in the medio-lateral direction. Representational changes in anterior-posterior direction were expressed by differences in polar angle $\Delta\varphi$ or by differences in eccentricity (Δr) and can be related to a change in source extent. Changes in the amount of cortical activity were examined by comparing the dipole strengths.

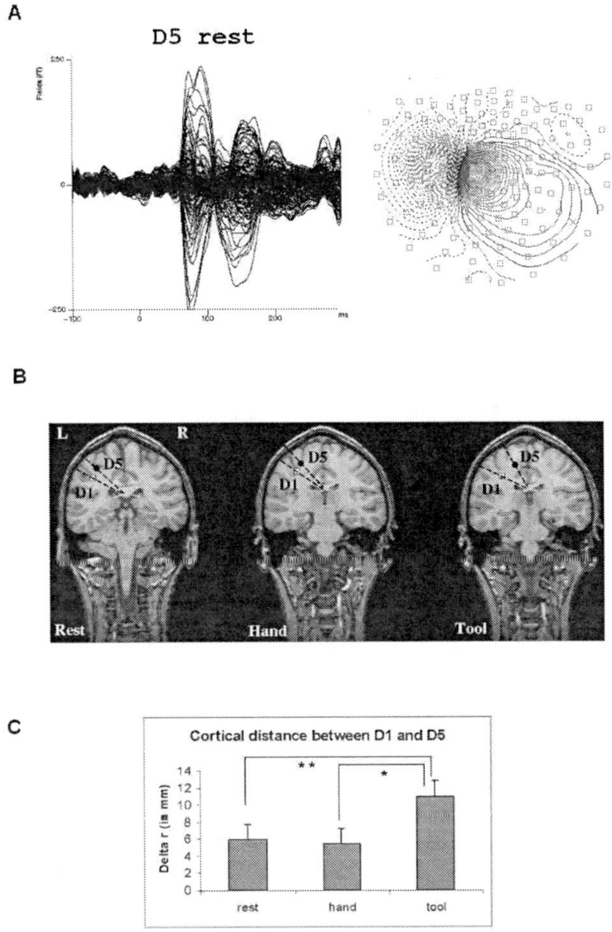

Figure 4. A: Topographic map and waveform of magnetic activity evoked by stimulation of the right D5 (single subject). Time courses of magnetic activity from 148 sensors are superimposed. Isocontour maps show the magnetic potential pattern elicited by stimulation of the right D5 at the first prominent peak after stimulus onset (nasion up, right side displays the right hemisphere, left side the left hemisphere). B: Neuromagnetic source localizations of the SEFs of D1 and D5 (results of one representative subject), overlaid onto a coronal MRI slice through the somatosensory cortex. The positions of the cortical representations of D5 and D1 are specified in polar coordinates. Note the differences between rest or hand condition and tool use condition, respectively. C: Mean differences of the cortical distance between the cortical representations of D1 and D5 during rest, hand

and tool condition. Asterisks indicate the significant differences between tool condition and rest, and tool condition and hand condition, respectively.

The resulting somatosensory magnetic fields revealed a clear dipolar topographic field pattern in the region over the central sulcus contralateral to the stimulated side (Figure 4). Neuromagnetic source imaging of these dipolar fields showed dipoles for the stimulated digits on the postcentral gyrus (SI). Further analysis (ANOVA and post-hoc t-tests) revealed that cortical representations of D1 and D5 were further apart during tool use as compared with the hand condition and baseline (Figure 3). Thus, tool use seems to change the functional organization of D1 and D5 in a very rapid way.

What is the meaning of the modulations in SI? Manipulation of small objects with tools is very familiar for humans, for example, while using spoons or forks or working with a screwdriver. Therefore, it seems to be improbable that a new sensory map is always acquired whenever this frequently executed task is performed. It is more likely that the somatosensory cortex switches between different concurrent pre-existing maps established earlier (Braun et al., 2001).

When an external object is used as a tool, it is felt as becoming a part or an extension of an arm or hand and thus incorporates the tool into body image. The results suggest that maps in SI are parts of the neural network representing the modified schema of the hand during tool use. Thus, the modified body schema during tool use seems not only involve the PPC but also SI and probably SII. Furthermore, the results demonstrate that the functional topography of SI can be modulated without preceding long-lasting sensory training or deafferentation.

Short-term plastic changes in SI as a result of top-down modulations have not only been reported as an effect of tool use. Other approaches show influences of the frontal lobe on somatosensory processing, thereby similarly demonstrating top-down processing. For example, Braun et al. (2002, see also Noppeneny et al., 1999) showed modulations of the functional organization of SI depending on the focus of attention. Subjects were trained to detect sequential leftward or rightward stimulus motion across the fingers of the left hand (hand condition) and in a different condition to detect stimulus motion at a specific finger on this hand (finger condition). Thus, the afferent input was identical for both conditions. The authors reported an increase of the distance between the cortical representations of the finger in the finger condition compared with the hand condition. Braun et al. (2002) concluded that the hand representation in SI is not fixed but can be dynamically altered by top-down mechanisms.

Further studies demonstrated rapid task-specific changes of the organization of SI as a result of motor activity. Braun et al. (2001) reported that the cortical representations of D1 and D5 were more distant during handwriting compared with rest in healthy humans. However, the results of the study were unable to distinguish whether these changes represented the consequence of altered reafferent input from joints, muscles and skin during the execution of the motor task or of a task-related influence of motor and premotor areas upon the organization of the somatosensory cortex. To test this hypothesis of a task-related influence of motor and premotor areas, we studied the functional topography of SI by examining coupling effects in a bimanual movement task (Schaefer et al., 2005a). Bimanual coupling is known to be related to an activation of the premotor cortex and the supplementary motor area (Sadato et al., 1997; Steyvers et al., 2003). The functional organization of the somatosensory cortex for known bimanual coupling effects was compared to the organization of the somatosensory cortex during the same movements but only with a small effort in coupling. More in detail, the blindfolded subjects were asked to produce cyclically trajectories with both hands. The direction of these trajectories was varied to be either the same (parallel) or different (orthogonal). In the parallel condition, the trajectories drawn by each hand were minimally affected in comparison to the performance of the hand alone. When they performed the movements in orthogonal direction (bimanual coupling task), trajectories deviated from their target paths (Franz et al., 1991; Franz, 1997, see also Figure 5). The kinematical displacements of the parallel and orthogonal movements were measured by quantifying the shape of the main drawn field. The widths of these drawings were computed for all conditions. We expected higher activation of the SMA and premotor cortex during the performing of the orthogonal task, because this task demands much higher bimanual coordination.

The subjects performed the tasks as expected. The trajectory of lines became elliptical when the other hand produced circles concurrently but not when the other hand produced lines like the dominant hand (Franz et al., 1991, see Figure 4). Results of neuromagnetic source imaging revealed that the neural sources of D1 and D5 moved further apart during the bimanual coupling task in comparison to the same task without coupling. This change correlated significantly positively with the displacement of the drawn lines during the orthogonal condition ($r = 0.69$; $p < 0.01$; Pearson correlation), suggesting dynamic modulations of SI as a result of a task-related influence of motor or premotor areas (see Figure 6).

This result suggests that cortical somatosensory representations not only depend on afferent input but also vary as a consequence of a possible task-related influence of motor or premotor areas. But how could neurons in the somatosensory cortex be affected by motor actions? Since SI has dense reciprocal connections with the motor cortex, Braun et al. (2001) as well as Schaefer et al.

(2004b, 2005a) suggested that feedback loops from these areas may explain these short-term plastic changes in SI.

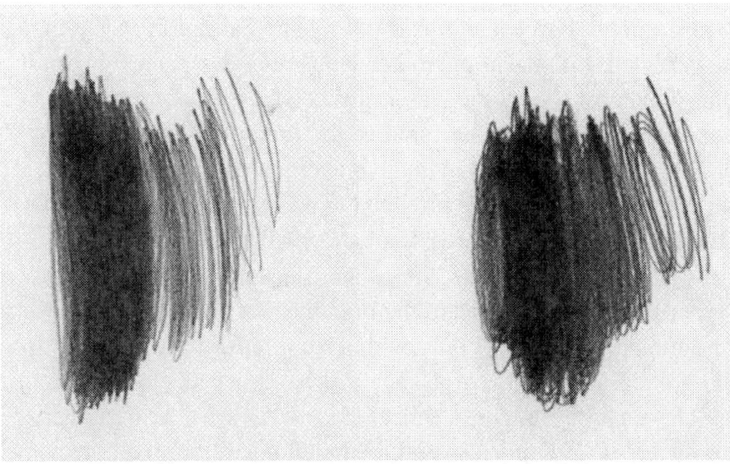

Figure 5. Typical displacement during the line task of the dominant hand when the other hand also produced lines (parallel condition, left side) and when the other hand produced circles (orthogonal condition, right side).

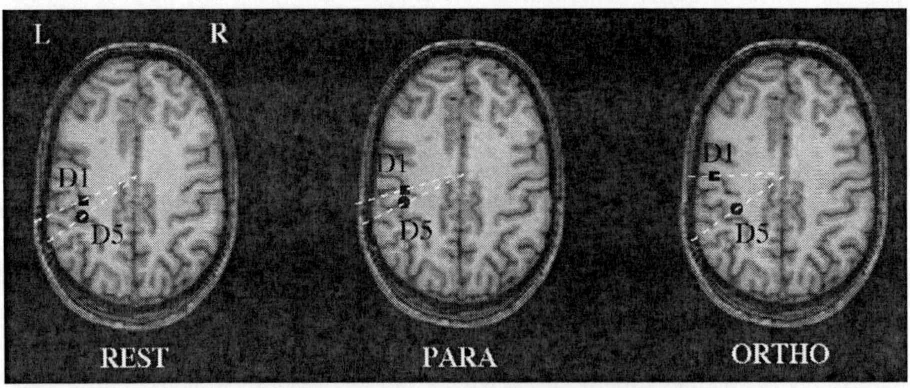

Figure 6. Source localization results of the somatosensory evoked fields of D1 (squares) and D5 (circles). Displayed are the results of one representative subject overlaid onto an axial MRI slice. Note the differences between rest or parallel condition (PARA) and orthogonal (ORTHO) condition.

Moreover, it has been proposed that a prefrontal-cortical sensory gating system may alter SI, depending on the requirements of different tasks (Staines et al., 2002). Staines et al. (2002) demonstrated that task-relevant somatosensory information leads to facilitation within the contralateral SI and to suppression of the ipsilateral SI. The authors showed that this modulation was associated with activation of the right prefrontal cortex, thereby demonstrating top-down influences of frontal areas on SI. Similar results have been reported by Chapman et al. (1988). Staines et al. (2002) concluded that there may be a prefrontal-cortical sensory gating system altering sensory information at the cortical level of SI to suit task-dependent needs for sensory inflow. Further, animal studies showed that the prefrontal cortex can regulate the flow of information to SI: Skinner and Yingling (1976) demonstrated the existence of a central gating mechanism in the brains of cats, which controlled sensory flow to primary cortical regions. These regulations were mediated by prefrontal-thalamic projections, which may provide a potential mechanism for suppressing irrelevant inputs and facilitating and selecting relevant ones (Guillery et al., 1998; McAlonan et al., 2000). In addition, studies with patients demonstrated that damage to the prefrontal cortex interrupts the ability to control sensory inputs in SI (Yamaguchi and Knight, 1990; Knight et al., 1999).

In a neuromagnetic study, we aimed to test this theory of a prefrontal-cortical sensory gating system (Schaefer et al., 2005b). Ten subjects participated in a task, which is known to rely on activation of frontal or prefrontal areas, and a comparable task involving the same movements but with no or only small contributions of frontal or prefrontal areas. The Tower of Hanoi task is a prototype task to study high-level cognition such as planning and problem-solving behavior (Simon, 1975). Studies with patients as well as imaging studies with healthy participants have shown that the neural mechanisms of the Tower of Hanoi task can be related to activation of frontal or prefrontal areas (Shallice, 1982; Anderson and Douglas, 2002). The Tower of Hanoi task used in our study consisted of three pegs and six discs forming a tower (all made of wood). The goal was to move all discs from the left peg to the right one. Only one disc might be moved at a time, and a disc could be placed either on an empty peg or on top of a larger disc. For the control task, subjects were asked to perform the same movements but with no specific task. Thus, subjects had to stockpile the rings in any type of order and to any cylinder, but with the same frequency of hand movements as in the Tower of Hanoi task.

Based on the theory of a prefrontal-cortical sensory gating system (Staines et al., 2002), we hypothesized that the pattern of activation of SI changes during the Tower of Hanoi task compared to the simple manual motor task, suggesting rapid modulation of cortical maps in SI.

A

B

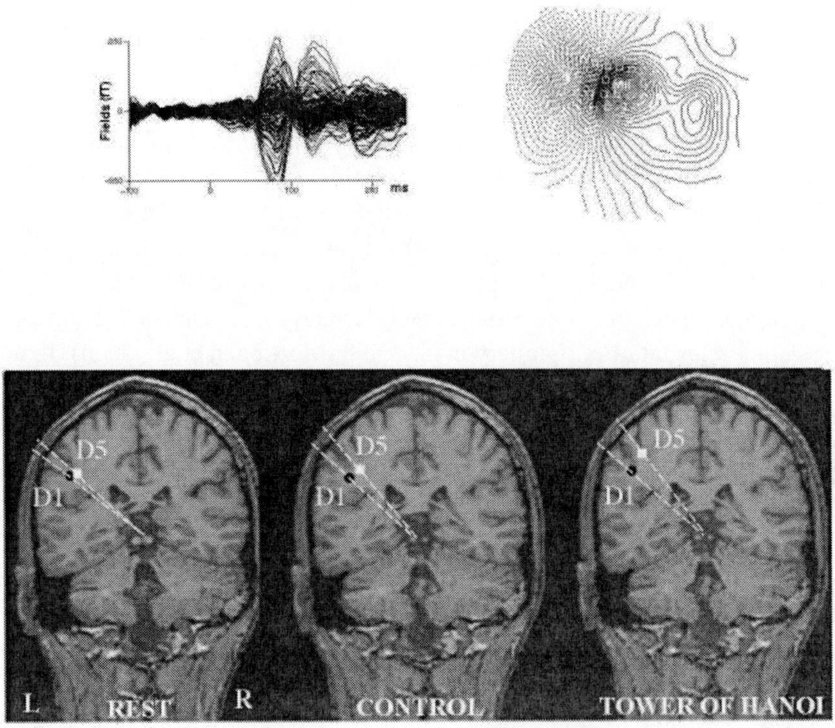

Figure 7. A: Neuromagnetic activity evoked by stimulation of D1 in a representative subject (rest condition). Isocontour maps show the magnetic potential pattern elicited by stimulation of the right D1 at the first prominent peak after stimulus onset (nasion up). B: Neuromagnetic source localizations of D1 and D5. Displayed are the results of one single representative subject overlaid onto a coronal MRI slice. Note the differences between rest, control task and Tower of Hanoi task.

More in detail, we expected an increased distance in the cortical representations of D1 and D5. Since previous work has demonstrated that this increase is associated with enhanced tactile perception (Elbert et al., 1995; Pleger et al., 2001), the results may thus provide evidence for a prefrontal-cortical sensory-gating system.

Neuromagnetic source imaging revealed effects of the task on the functional topography in SI. When subjects performed the Tower of Hanoi task, the cortical representations of D1 and D5 moved further apart compared to the control task containing the same movements but without the cognitive characteristic (see Figure 7). Thus, performing motor tasks with different cognitive demands results in a dynamic modulation of SI. The results provide support for a prefrontal-cortical sensory-gating system, which means that frontal or prefrontal areas can facilitate neuronal responsiveness in SI according to different task demands. Since it is known that shifts of the cortical representations of the finger along the postcentral gyrus can be related to an increased tactile perception (Pleger et al., 2001), the results are able to relate this modulation of SI to a prefrontal-cortical sensory-gating system.

What is the implication of these shifts in SI? It seems to be unlikely that a new sensory map is learned whenever this motor task is performed (see above for tool use). Similar to tool use, bimanual coordination of skilled finger movements is a frequent applied task for humans. Braun et al. (2001) suggested that specific representational maps may be activated by dynamically switching between stable maps established earlier, depending on actual task requirements. Nicolelis and Fanselow (2002) provided further evidence to this interpretation by showing that the physiological properties of thalamic neurons in the ventral posterior medial nucleus in rats shift between different behavioral states, which consist of distinct modes of rhythmic whisker movements. This dynamic switching of somatosensory maps might be related to sub-threshold synaptic activities (Moore and Nelson, 1998). The task-specific activations of concurrently preexisting maps within a certain representational zone may represent a general principle to optimize stimulus processing (Braun et al., 2001).

Chapter 4

SI REPRESENTS THE PERCEIVED RATHER THAN THE PHYSICAL IMAGE OF THE BODY

When Penfield and Boldrey (1937) described the somatosensory homunculus, they proposed a body map that was not only supposed to be fixed but also was considered as representing the physical image of the body in a relatively mechanical way. As shown above, recent research has questioned this view and suggests a much more complex role for SI in establishing and maintaining a first image of the body. Thus, plastic changes in the topography of SI may occur after amputation of a limb. Further, short-term modulations of the cortical representations of the finger have been reported depending on tool use, task related, or on the focus of attention. Moreover, some studies suggest that the topography in SI is not only adapting to different situational requirements but represents the *perception* of tactile stimulation rather than the physical location of touch delivered to the body. Thus, the somatosensory homunculus may code a first image of the body based on the perceived situation of the received touch, in contrast to the mere reflection of physical stimulation in a mechanical way.

An important experiment providing support for this hypothesis is reported in an animal study by Chen et al. (2003). The authors were interested in the role of the somatosensory cortex during the tactile funneling illusion. The funneling illusion consists of a simultaneous stimulation of two points on the skin, which produces a single focal sensation at the center of the stimulus pattern, even when no physical stimulus occurs at that site. Chen et al. (2003) used the technique of optical imaging to examine the role of SI (Area 3b) in monkeys during this illusion. They reported that simultaneous stimulation of two fingertips produced a single focal cortical activation located between the expected regions for each single fingertip activation. Thus, the authors concluded that the topographic organization in SI reflects the *perceived* rather than the physical location of peripheral stimulation.

Further evidence came from subsequent studies with human subjects. Using fMRI, Blankenburg et al. (2006) similarly examined a somatosensory illusion that can dissociate tactile perception from physical stimulation. The so-called cutaneous rabbit illusion consists of repeated rapid stimulation at the wrist followed by the skin near the elbow. This procedure evokes the illusion of touches at intervening locations along the arm, as if a rabbit hopped along it. FMRI results revealed that illusory sequences activated contralateral SI at a somatotopic location corresponding to the filled-in illusory perception on the forearm (compared with a control condition). The authors concluded that illusory somatosensory perception affected SI. Moreover, the results demonstrated that this activation was somatotopically organized, providing further support for our hypothesis.

The understanding that the functional topography in SI may reflect the perceived shape of the body rather than physical aspects of peripheral stimulation was further supported by neuromagnetic studies on multisensory integration. It has been long established that vision often dominates the tactile modality (e.g., Rock and Victor, 1964). Thus, simple manipulations of multisensory integration may result in tactile illusions (e.g., Ramachandran and Rogers-Ramachandran, 1996; Ramachandran, 1998). In order to test the hypothesis that brain activity at early stages of sensory processing is susceptible for tactile illusions, we created an experiment to evoke the illusion of a referred sensation while examining neuromagnetic activity in SI (Schaefer et al., 2006a).

We mentioned the astonishing phenomenon of referred sensations above in the chapter about phantom sensations. After the amputation of a limb, many patients not only experience painful phantom sensations but also referred sensations. These referred sensations are felt in their phantoms and can be triggered by certain points on the body, e.g., the cheek or the shoulder, sometimes even in a topographic manner (Ramachandran, 1998). However, Ramachandran and Hirstein (1998) also discuss tactile illusions in healthy subjects that resemble phantom phenomena in amputees. These illusions can be induced by simple manipulations of sensory and visual information.

Here, we were interested in an illusion of a referral of a somatic sensation on the same body surface. Hence, we tried to induce a referred sensation in healthy individuals similar to that reported in phantom-limb patients. While recording their brain activity with MEG, subjects watched a video that showed a hand that was stroked by a stick on D1 while actually receiving real tactile stimuli on D5.

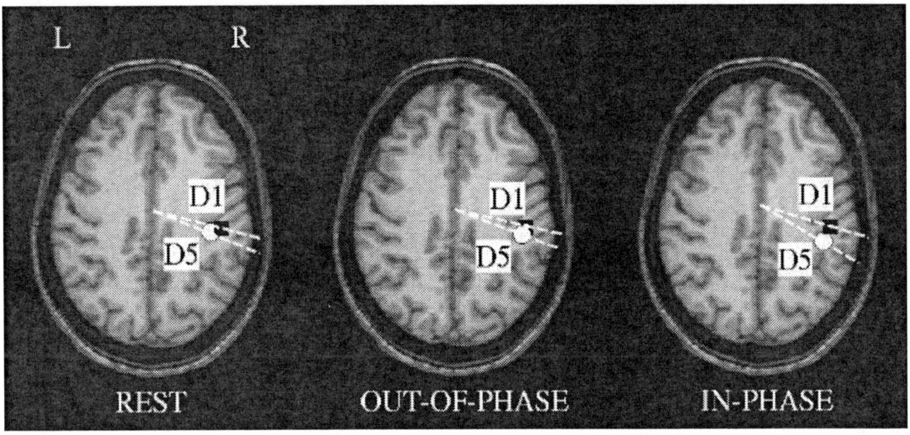

Figure 8. Results of the neuromagnetic source imaging. Differences between D1 and D5 demonstrate an increase of source extent of the dipole source of D5 in the experimental condition (in-phase).

The video was presented in the peripersonal space of the subject at a distance where the real hand would be expected. Thus, we created an experimental conflict between tactile and visual senses. Due to the known dominance of the visual modality over somatosensation (Rock and Victor, 1964), we hypothesized that the participants would feel the stroking on D1 instead of D5. Therefore, we described this tactile illusion as an artificially induced referred sensation. Moreover, we hypothesized that SI is prone to this kind of tactile illusions. When the topographic organization in SI reflects the perceived rather than the physical location of peripheral stimulation, the functional topography should be affected by the illusion.

Results revealed that subjects indeed felt the illusion of being touched on D1 instead of D5. Neuromagnetic source imaging based on tactile stimulation with a pneumatic stimulator (analogous to our previous MEG experiments) revealed that this tactile illusion was accompanied by changes in the topography of the functional organization of SI (see Figure 8). The cortical representation of D5 shifted towards a more posterior location, pointing to an enlargement of the cortical representation. Moreover, the amount of the referred sensation was significantly correlated with the modulation in SI: The more the subjects felt the illusion of being touched on the thumb (instead of the actually stimulated pinky), the more SI was modulated. Thus, the results confirmed that in contrast to traditional views of the body map, the topographic representation in SI reflects the perceived rather than the physical location of peripheral stimulation. Further, these findings demonstrate that not only tactile illusions based on modulations in the tactile modality (e.g., the funneling illusion or the cutaneous rabbit illusion) may alter the somatosensory topography, but also tactile illusions based on manipulations of multisensory integration. Hence, the results point to multisensory processing in SI, an area of the brain that long has been regarded as being strictly unimodal.

Why was the cortical representation of D5 moved to a more posterior position when subjects felt an illusory touch? Classical studies demonstrated that there are several digit representations in the parietal lobe (area 3b, 1, 2, 5) (e.g., Kaas et al., 1979). Areas 3a and 2 of the somatosensory cortices have dense reciprocal connections with the motor system and the PPC, in which bimodal neurons were found. Feedback from these areas may have influenced somatosensory processing. Area 2 has connections with the rostral part of the PPC that receives visual input from the more caudal parts of the PPC. This might have potentiated activity in area 2 in this study, resulting in the posterior shift of D5.

Inducing a conflict between vision and intention of movements, Fink et al. (1999) reported an activation of a right dorsolateral prefrontal cortex area whenever the visual feedback contradicted the intended movements. According to Harris (1999), this area might be the anatomical correlate for the perceived incongruence between proprioception, visual feedback and motor intention. Harris suggested that this area may also be involved in phantom-limb pain, focal dystonia and nausea. However, one could speculate that there might be an analogue area in the parietal lobe for the perceived incongruence between proprioception, visual feedback and tactile information, which was subject of manipulation in our study. This area may be located in the PPC, which may have altered the topography in SI via feedback-loops.

It remains unclear if the tactile illusion of a referred sensation reported in the last study is based on similar neural circuits or referred sensations known in patients with phantom limbs. The observation that phantom sensations could be evoked from the intact and the amputated side (pointing to an involvement of SII) as well as from distal areas (Grüsser et al., 2004) and the fact that there is cortical reorganization not only in SI (Flor et al., 1995) but also in the thalamus (Jones and Pons, 1998) and motor cortex (Karl et al., 2001), seem to point to a multifactorial model of the origin of phantom limbs.

Chapter 5

THE TWO-FOLD CHARACTER OF TOUCH: VIEWING THE BODY MAGNIFIED

Touch is different from other senses. When we feel touch, we receive information at the same time about the external object touching the skin as well as about the body itself (Serino and Haggard, 2009). Although we are aware of this interdependence of body and touch, little is known about this interaction. Here, we review some experiments that manipulate this interaction, thereby proposing a model of a dynamic body representation in SI.

The perception of the body is based in particular on visual and tactile senses, which have to be integrated to produce a coherent internal representation. In the traditional understanding, the role of SI is to be a first major unimodal area processing somatosensory input. However, increasing evidence suggests cross-modal links between vision and somatosensation even at this early stage of sensory processing. An important finding has been reported by Kennett et al. (2001). Using behavioral experiments, they revealed that subjects were more accurate in detecting invisible tactile stimuli when they were looking at their stimulated body parts compared to viewing a neutral object presented at the same location. Hence, viewing the body can improve tactile acuity. Moreover, this so-called visual enhancement of touch was best when the visual appearance of the arm was magnified.

The neural correlates of these cross-modal interactions remain unclear. Previous studies found neurons in the monkey parietal and premotor cortex, which respond both to tactile and visual stimuli (e.g., Graziano et al., 1994, 2000; Iriki et al., 1996). Recent evidence suggests that some neurons in SI can code arbitrary visuo-tactile associations: Animal studies have shown that neurons in monkey SI may fire both in response to a tactile stimulus and also in response to a visual stimulus previously associated with the tactile stimulus (Zhou and Fuster, 1997). Some of these neurons even showed sustained activity during the visuo-tactile delay period (Zhou and Fuster, 2000). Based on those studies, Kennett et al. (2001) suggested that the neural correlates for the visual enhancement effects may correspond to modulations in SI, probably induced by back projections from multimodal cortical areas.

First evidence for this hypothesis was provided by an experiment of Taylor-Clarke et al. (2002). The authors used EEG to examine activity in SI in a visuo-tactile enhancement experiment where they manipulated the visibility of the arm and also used a neutral object as a further control condition. Taylor-Clarke et al. (2002) could demonstrate altered somatosensory potentials associated with the known effects of the visual enhancement of touch in a two-point-tactile-discrimination task. However, although this study successfully linked the behavioral improvements with modulations in SI when seeing the body being touched, it remains unclear if the effects for seeing a *magnified* body part are similarly based on alterations in SI.

To further examine the role of SI while seeing the own stimulated body part in different ways, we conducted an MEG study (Schaefer et al., 2008a). According to the original experiment of Kennett et al. (2001), we compared the topography of SI in a resting state, while seeing the stimulated hand, and while viewing a neutral object of comparable size. The last condition was added to control for spatial attention and gaze-direction effects. Furthermore, we varied the size of the seen body part and presented it in real size or strongly magnified.

For delivering tactile stimulation, we used the established pneumatical stimulation device to the index (D2) and little finger (D5) of the participants while employing neuromagnetic source localization to map the cortical representations of these fingers. Tactile stimuli were applied at the distal phalanges of D2 and D5 of the left hand. The stimulation device was identical to the one we used in the previous studies. It consisted of a diaphragm with a 10-mm diameter, causing a distinct tactile sensation when inflated toward the skin by a pulse of pressed air of 2.5 atm for 20 ms. Subjects could easily observe the tactile stimulation on their fingers when the hand was shown on a screen via a video camera in the peripersonal space of the subjects, close to the area where the real hand was placed (see Figure 3). Since the room was acoustically shielded, the participants were not able to hear any sounds associated with the pneumatical stimulation device.

Results confirmed the hypothesis of Kennett et al. (2001) and Taylor-Clarke et al. (2002) by demonstrating modulations in SI when seeing the own hand being touched compared with control conditions. Statistical tests revealed that the cortical representation of the observed digit shifted to a more superior position when its stimulation could be observed via the screen (compared with control and baseline conditions). Further, we found that the magnification of the seen stimulated hand similarly resulted in dynamic alterations of the somatosensory homunculus (Figure 9). When the stimulated digit could be observed magnified, its cortical representation shifted to a more superior position compared to a resting state without any visual information of the stimulated digit.

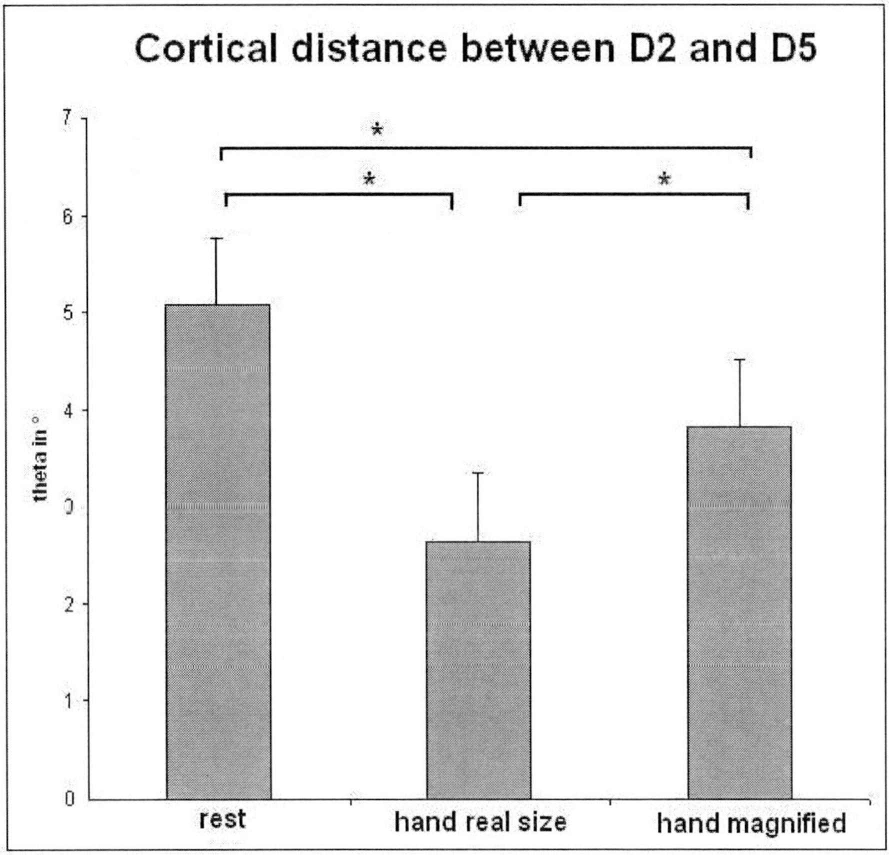

Figure 9. Results of the neuromagnetic source imaging. Bars represent group means for the cortical distance between D2 and D5. Asterisks indicate significant differences between the conditions "observe hand magnified" and "observe hand in real size" and rest, respectively.

Thus, the results demonstrate that visibility of tactile stimulation can change the functional organization in SI. Integration of visual and tactile information, necessary to form a representation of peripersonal space, seems to engage brain areas like SI, which was previously thought to be strictly unimodal. This is in line with previous studies pointing to dynamic interactions between vision and touch (e.g., Rock and Victor, 1964; Taylor-Clarke et al., 2002; Ro et al., 2004). The present study extends those previous results by showing that watching the touched body part *magnified* affects SI compared to viewing it in real size or to a rest state.

Why is there a shift in the somatosensory homunculus when subjects view their stimulated hands and why is there a further modulation when they see their hands magnified? Due to the nature of shift (along the postcentral gyrus), an extension of the sensory cortical representation seems to be unlikely (Braun et al., 2001). Similar to the studies discussed above, we think that different concurrent pre-existing maps in SI may exist. The organization of the somatosensory cortex may then switch between those pre-existing maps according to specific task requirements in familiar situations. This rapid remapping may be based on feedback projections from multimodal areas such as the PPC or premotor cortex. Lifelong experiences of touch when viewing the hand and when not seeing it may possibly have resulted in this kind of different concurrent maps in SI.

But why is the visual magnification of the hand leading to a shift in somatosensory cortex? The somatosensory homunculus represents tactile information through a distorted representation of the body surface. On the one hand, this distorted organization allows improved representation of important body parts like the mouth or fingers. On the other hand, it raises the problem of maintaining perceptual constancy (Taylor-Clarke et al., 2004). Using a magnified view of the arm, Taylor-Clarke et al. (2004) demonstrated that tactile stimuli are rescaled to the visually specified physical size of body parts in order to achieve tactile object constancy. The results of this study similarly varied the view of a stimulated hand from normal size to strongly magnified. Since the results showed an altered functional organization of the somatosensory cortex when viewing the hand magnified (compared with normal size and rest), we speculate that these rescaling processes (Taylor-Clarke et al., 2004) may be reflected by an altered map in SI. Again, these modulations may be based on different concurrent preexisting defined maps (Braun et al., 2001). Thus, the modulation in SI associated with the visual magnification of the stimulated body part we reported here may be linked to rescaling processes. Since the brain attempts to keep tactile object perception in a constant size, the visually distorted view of the body part must be rescaled. This process may involve changes in SI.

In our study, we reported that observing a touched hand is associated with modulations in SI. Since we only measured the cortical representations of D2, we cannot state how specific this effect is. Thus, it remains unclear if the reported modulations are limited to the cortical representation of D2 or if they can be generalized to the representation of the whole hand. Furthermore, the reported modulation must not necessarily be limited to SI of one hemisphere but may also affect the ipsilateral SI. Future studies are necessary to clarify these questions.

While previous studies have shown that observing touch on the own body enhances tactile sensitivity, the results of our experiment together with the outcome of the study of Taylor-Clarke et al. (2002) demonstrate that this visual-tactile enhancement probably relies at least in part on SI. Moreoever, further support is provided by a recent study relating shifts of cortical representations along the postcentral gyrus with human discrimination improvement (Pleger et al., 2001). However, from the above-mentioned studies, it remains unclear if the simple view of the body part is crucial for the visuo-tactile enhancement or if viewing the *touch* is more important, which may be imagined by the subjects in the classic studies on visuo-tactile enhancement (e.g., Kennett et al., 2001).

In order to test this, we conducted a behavioral study in which we varied the visual information by presenting a tactile stimulated body part in the experimental condition and showed the same body part without any tactile stimulation in a control condition (Schaefer et al., 2005c). Participants were instructed to watch a video showing a hand being touched by a stick (touch video, experimental condition) and a second video showing the same hand and stick, but this time the stick touched the space (nontouch video, control condition). Thus, the visual stimuli as well as the motion components were kept constant. Before and after each movie, sensory thresholds were tested with von-Frey-filaments on the index fingers of both hands. Based on previous studies (Ro et al.2004; Rock and Victor, 1964), we assumed that observation of tactile stimulation improves tactile threshold on the stimulated body part more than observation of a just depicted hand.

An ANOVA for changes of the tactile threshold revealed a significant interaction effect for condition and location. Post hoc t-tests showed a significant improvement of the tactile threshold of the right index finger after the "touch" video but not after the "no touch" video. For the left index finger, which was not presented in the videos, no significant effects were obtained (see Figure 10).

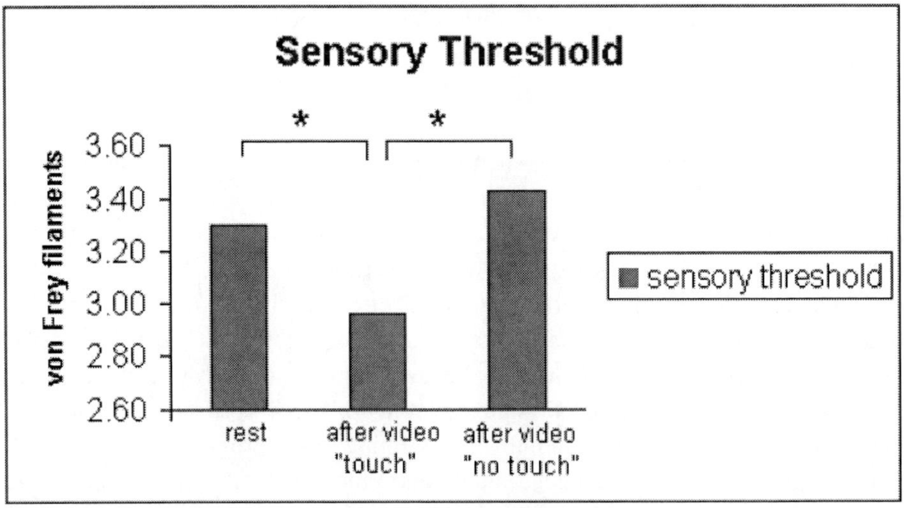

Figure 10. Sensory threshold for the index finger before (rest state) and after the different videos. In the "touch" video, a hand where the index finger was touched with a stick was shown. In the "no touch" video, the same hand and stick were shown, but the stick did not hit the index finger but rather the space beneath the finger. Asterisks indicate a significance increase of sensory threshold after the observing touch video.

The results demonstrated that only after viewing the video that showed the hand being touched, the sensory threshold improves significantly. When subjects were presented with a movie showing the same hand and stick and also the same motion of the stick but lacking a touch the hand, no significant improvement of the sensory threshold occurred. In addition, this improvement was specific only for the index finger, which was presented in the video; the index finger of the other hand showed no improvement. Thus, it seems that observation of *touch* but not simply depicting the stimulated body part improves tactile perception measured as tactile threshold with von-Frey-filaments. Furthermore, this improvement of tactile perception was demonstrated several minutes after presenting the visual stimuli.

The results extend previous outcomes by suggesting that the observation of *touch* (and not of a mere body part) is crucial for the visuo-tactile enhancement. Moreover, this visuo-tactile enhancement seemed to last several minutes and was linked only to the index finger shown in the video. Hence, the visuo-tactile enhancement seems closely related to the cognitive content of the movie and not to the mere picture of the body part.

Why is there an increased sensitivity of touch after a simple observation of a tactile stimulation persisting even minutes after the video and no effect after watching a similar video that is lacking to touch the video hand? Visuo-tactile associations seem to be very common in everyday life. The touch of a hand often occurs when both the tactile stimulus and the hand can be seen, hence forming a visual-tactile association. We speculate that those visual-tactile associations may improve somatosensory functions (sensory gating). Zhou et al. (1997) have shown that neurons in SI respond to visual stimuli when they have been previously associated with touch. Some of these neurons even showed activity over a time delay (2000). These results may suggest a cross-modal temporary memory in SI (Wheeler et al., 2000). Several neuropsychological studies demonstrated that vision of a deafferented limb might improve the somatosensory abilities, pointing to a mechanism that binds together tactile and visual stimuli within the peripersonal space (e.g., Di Pellegrino et al., 1997). In addition, a recent case study reported that vision of the workspace adjacent to the unseen hand is sufficient to enhance somatosensory information of the unseen hand (Newport et al., 2001). The results of the present study extend these data by showing that visuo-tactile associations can be induced simply by observing touch, and these associations or memory traces can be recalled up to several minutes after the presentation.

In the present study, the video hand appeared in the same position as the subject's real hand. From the results of this experiment, it remains unclear if the exposition of the visual stimuli in the peripersonal space is necessary for the effect and if the increase of tactile enhancement will disappear when presenting the video hand outside of the peripersonal space. Using a rubber hand, Pavani and colleagues (2000) showed that visual information about the apparent hand position can influence tactile perception. Future studies may examine if the location (close to the real hand) and position of the video hand (first-person perspective) are necessary for the increase of tactile sensitivity reported in our study.

Our results suggest that a simple observational training can establish visuo-tactile associations that may lead to an increased tactile performance for several minutes after presenting the visual stimuli. These results are also supported by studies that have demonstrated that action observation combined with physical practice results in more prominent training effects relative to plain training effects. This has been reported in healthy volunteers (Stefan et al., 2005; Celnik et al., 2006) as well as in patients with chronic stroke (Celnik et al., 2008), suggesting that this facilitory process is of potential high value for neurorehabilitation. More specifically, Celnik et al. (2006) could show that observation of motor training alone improved the formation of a motor memory, but the combination of an observation of a motor training combined with doing the same movement on their own resulted in the best results regarding the effect of building a motor memory. Thus, the results provide congruent effects for the motor domain, as we have seen for the tactile sense. We speculate that boosting somatosensory functions simply by a short observational training may have important clinical implications for patients with somatosensory impairments (Rorden et al. 1999; Sathian et al. 1999).

In contrast to Kennett et al. (2001), Celnik et al. (2006, 2008) try to explain their results in a different way. While Kennett et al. (2001) label their effect visuo-tactile enhancement, Celnik et al. (2006,2008) link their results to the mirror neuron system theory (Rizzolatti et al., 2001), assuming that observing another individual performing actions activates mirror neurons in premotor and parietal areas as well as in the primary motor cortex (M1). However, the crucial difference is if subjects observe their own bodies, as in the visuo-tactile enhancement experiments, or if they observe the body of someone else. Only in the latter condition, an involvement of a mirror neuron system seems to make sense (as we will see in the next chapters). We do not know if the subjects in the motor tasks tend to imagine that the seen practicing hand is their own or if they believed that this hand belonged to the body of someone else, pointing to a real observation of an action. Moreover, it remains an open question why and how the mirror neurons may contribute to an improvement in motor or somatosensory functions.

Chapter 6

MORPHING THE BODY

"One morning, as Gregor Samsa was waking up from anxious dreams, he discovered that in bed, he had been changed into a monstrous verminous bug. He lay on his armour-hard back and saw, as he lifted his head up a little, his brown, arched abdomen divided up into rigid bow-like sections. From this height, the blanket, just about ready to slide off completely, could hardly stay in place. His numerous legs, pitifully thin in comparison to the rest of his circumference, flickered helplessly before his eyes. 'What's happened to me,' he thought. It was no dream."

This is the beginning of the famous novel *The Metamorphosis* by Franz Kafka, in which the hero suddenly awakes with the body of a bug, including a huge appetite for rotten apples and similar "food." Kafka's work used this metamorphosis as a metaphor to describe how odd we sometimes feel in our bodies and lives. And, indeed, we all sometimes feel a little bit displaced in our bodies, like an ugly bug whose thoughts and feelings nobody understands, and we all want to get rid of or to be changed into a more "normal" person.

Bodily transformations or malformations are a popular topic in literature and movies. Think, for example, of Joseph Carey Merrick (1862-1890), an Englishman who became known as the "Elephant Man" because of his physical appearance caused by a congenital defect. His life was the subject of many books, plays, and movies. Another famous work based on body transformation is *Frankenstein* or, the Modern Prometheus by Mary Shelley. As we probably all known, this novel is about a scientist named Frankenstein, who learned how to create life and forms a powerful and huge being in the likeness of man. In the tradition of this work, many other books and movies used similar stories. One example may be the work by David Cronenberg, whose movies often deal with themes of bodily disfigurement or metamorphosis. Also contemporary artists work with transformed bodies or bodies that are partly artificial. The American artist Cindy Sherman has been getting very popular by using these topics. When watching an exhibition by Cindy Sherman, the visitor often is warned that the presented pictures might be offending for some people. Considering that those potentially offending pictures only display puppets, the warning seems to be almost ridiculous. However, when we actually see those pictures of puppets in different situations, we really feel touched by them, although we know and easily can see that these images depict puppets and not humans. So why are we affected so easily by anthropomorphic stories or depictions, even when we know that they are artificial or fictional and, for example, just part of an art project? This chapter will try to provide some evidence that even early stages of sensory processing are involved in the perception of bodies and body distortions. The early time of processing this bodily information may perhaps at least partly explain why we so easily feel "touched" when we are faced with anthropomorphic depictions or stories.

The above-mentioned studies have shown that the body map in SI seems to adapt dynamically to different situational requirements. In particular, they have shown that the functional topography in SI reflects the perceived rather than the physical location of peripheral stimulation (see chapter 4). The experiments that led to this conclusion were based on tactile illusions, for example, on manipulations of multisensory integration (Schaefer et al., 2006a). However, recent studies also suggest that we do not necessarily need to create an illusion to affect the functional organization in SI. It seems sufficient to change the visual appearance or shape of the body to modestly distort our feeling of our own bodies. Moreover, this altered body perception was accompanied with corresponding modulations in the topography of SI. Thus, simply viewing the body "disguised" may elicit feelings of a morphed body, associated with changes in the somatosensory homunculus. Two studies provide evidence for this view.

In a first study, we manipulated the visual information about the subject's body to elicit the appearance of an elongated arm (Schaefer et al., 2007). For this purpose, we used an artificial hand and arm, which were attached in an anatomically correct way over the subject's real hand and arm and connected to the body of the participant. Therefore, subjects had to wear a shirt over their left arms, which was prepared in a way that the sleeve appeared longer (about 20 cm). At the end of this sleeve of the left arm, part of an artificial arm and hand were attached. The artificial body part was made of rubber. Thus, subjects viewed their arms as extended by about 20 cm (Figure 11).

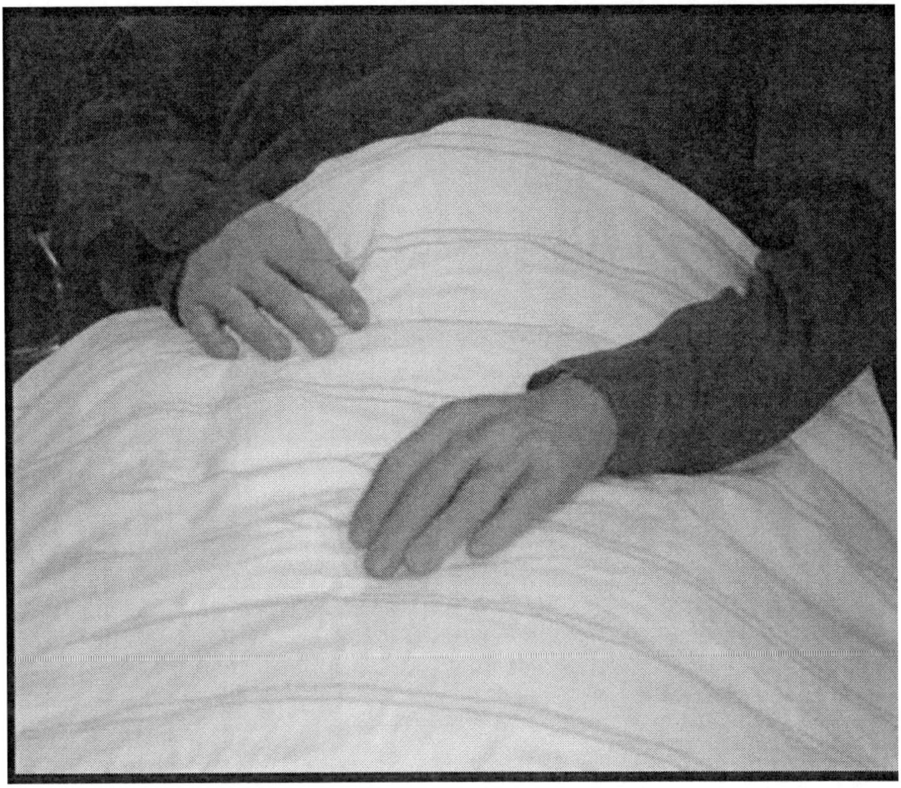

Figure 11. Experimental condition of elongated arm. The artificial hand and arm in front is attached to the subject's body by the use of a special shirt. The subject is seeing his arm elongated by about a length of 20 cm.

As a control condition, we presented the same artificial hand and arm close to the body of the subjects, but did not connect them to their bodies. Since it is known that the visual sense often dominates the tactile modality (Rock and Victor, 1964), we hypothesized that subjects would modestly feel the elongated arm when the artificial arm was connected to their bodies (compared with control conditions).

To examine the role of SI in this illusion, we recorded neuromagnetic fields related to the stimulation of D5 and D1. Since the cortical representation of the upper or lower arm in SI is relatively small and difficult to measure, we used the representations of D1 and D5 to determine dynamic modulations in SI in an indirect way. We assumed that the illusion of an elongated arm would affect the topography in SI, providing support of our hypothesis that SI is adapting dynamically to different situational requirements and that it is reflecting the perceived rather than the actual body shape.

The results of a questionnaire indicated that the participants not only viewed their arms as elongated, but also *felt* this arm extended. In the illusion condition, five of the subjects claimed to have a strong feeling that their left arms were elongated (four to six on a six-point scale). Neuromagnetic source imaging of the functional organization in SI revealed that the illusion was accompanied by shifts in the cortical distance between D1 and D5 (see Figure 12). These modulations were significantly correlated with the feeling of an extended arm (Spearman's rho, r = 0.59): the more the subjects felt the illusion, the smaller was the distance of the cortical representations of D1 and D5. Thus, the results suggest an involvement of SI in perceived changes in the size of body parts.

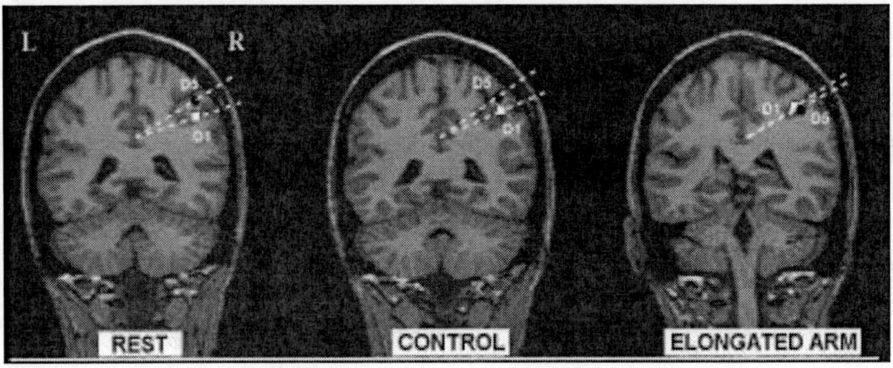

Figure 12. Dipole solutions of the SEFs of D5 (circles) and D1 (squares) overlaid onto a coronal MRI slice. Note the differences for the cortical representations between rest or control condition and elongated arm condition.

The illusion of an elongated arm was accompanied with a decrease of the distance between the representation zones of D1 and D5. How exactly is this cortical shift related to the illusion? We speculate that this representational change might be an indirect effect of an enlargement of the representation zone of the arm, which appears longer in the illusion condition. Since the subjects in the illusion suddenly felt that their arms were longer than usual, the cortical representation zone of the arm may have been grown to represent this now bigger arm. Given that the cortical representation of the arm is located above the representation of the hand in the somatosensory homunculus, the cortical representation of D5 may have been "pushed" into an inferior position as a result of the increased arm representation. However, since we did not measure changes of the cortical representation of the lower arm (or the upper arm, which is located above the lower arm in the homunculus) directly, this explanation remains speculative. Nevertheless, recent studies demonstrated enhanced tactile performance just because of a magnification of the seen body part (Kennett et al. 2001), whereby this visual enhancement of touch seems to be linked to SI (Taylor-Clarke et al., 2002; Schaefer et al., 2008a) and might be based on an enlargement of representational zones.

The results suggest that the perception of the size or shape of one's own body involves dynamic modulations in SI. We interpret the results as reflecting feedback loops from higher somatosensory areas, e.g., the PPC. For instance, the IPS contains cells that have complex receptive fields including several body parts (Mountcastle, 1959) or bilateral receptive fields. Increased activity in the IPS due to the necessary recalibration of body size and shape may have affected the topography in SI, resulting in a shift of the cortical representation of the hand. Similar local changes from multimodal to unimodal areas due to top-down feedback have been reported in the visual cortex of monkeys (Driver and Spence, 2000; Rockland and Ojima, 2003).

Although we think that higher cortical areas (containing bimodal neurons) might have had an influence on SI in this kind of illusion, we do not think that the modulation of the map in SI was just a simple reflection of these higher areas. The results of this study together with other recent work on body perception (e.g., Ehrsson et al., 2006) suggest that the body image might be based on a network of different cortical areas, which play different functional roles in maintaining a coherent and dynamic image of the body. What exactly might be the role for SI in this network? Since SI is an important early area in the processing of somatosensory stimuli, it may provide a first dynamic and transient coherent image of the body by using tactile and also visual (from other cortical areas) information.

Similar to the study reported above, Ehrsson et al. (2005) described an illusion of perceived changes in the size of body parts. Ehrsson et al. (2005) used an experimental illusion described by Lackner (1988; Goodwin et al., 1972). In a fascinating study, Lackner (1988) used this paradigm to evoke the "Pinocchio illusion." The blindfolded subject was sitting at a table with his or her arm flexed at the elbow and holding the tip of his or her own nose, while the experimenter was using a vibrator to stimulate the tendon of the biceps. As a result of this manipulation, the subject was not only feeling that his or her arm was extended, but also that his or her nose was lengthened. Thus, the participant was feeling like Pinocchio. Ehrsson et al. (2005) used this approach to elicit the illusory feeling of shrinking of the waist and examined the brain regions involved with this shrinking illusion with fMRI. The results revealed activity in the postcentral gyrus and also in the anterior part of the IPS that was correlated with the degree of the illusion. However, although Ehrsson et al. reported activity in the anterior parietal cortex, they did not find any activity in SI. The lack of activity might be related to the different kind of body size change (shrinking waist vs. elongated arm), or due to the different body part (waist vs. arm), but the most important difference seems to be the employed technique. Whereas Ehrsson et al. used a manipulation of proprioception and somatosensation to evoke the illusion, the illusion we used was based on a manipulation of the visual modality.

A second study in our lab used even more dramatic manipulations of the visual appearance of the participants. The experiment aimed to extend the hypothesis that the somatosensory homunculus mirrors the phenomenally perceived shape of the body by investigating if even artificial supernumerary body parts may be represented in the somatosensory homunculus when being illusory felt.

In order to test this, subjects were given the visual impression that they had a supernumerary third arm and hand (Schaefer et al., 2008b). Participants were asked to wear a special shirt with an artificial third arm between both of their own arms. This third artificial rubbery arm ended in front of the original arms. Hence, the participants viewed this artificial hand and arm connected to their bodies between the left arm and the middle of their bodies (see Figure 13). In a control condition, the artificial hand and arm were put in front of the subjects. Hence, subjects could see the artificial hand and arm close to their bodies, but the artificial body parts were not connected to their bodies.

Due to the known dominance of the visual modality (Rock and Victor, 1964; Schaefer et al., 2007), we hypothesized that the subjects would not only view the third arm but more or less would feel this third arm and transiently believe that this hand and arm belong to their own bodies. Furthermore, since we assumed that even artificial body parts that were illusory felt might be represented in the somatosensory homunculus, we expected alterations in SI related to this illusory feeling.

Results revealed that most of the participants at least transiently reported the sensation of feeling the third arm. This feeling was associated with modulations in SI (Figure 14). Neuromagnetic source imaging revealed that the cortical representation of D1 was shifting to a more medial and superior position on the somatosensory cortex when subjects felt the illusion. Moreover, the amount of this shift predicted the strength of the illusion. Thus, the somatosensory homunculus seems to mirror the perceived shape of the body rather than physical aspects of peripheral stimulation, even when feeling an artificial additional body part. The reason for this shift may be that the "new" third hand might be located directly below the cortical representation of D1, resulting in a shift towards a more medial and superior position of the representation for D1. We concluded that the perceived body image in SI is not only prone to tactile illusions on the body surface but also can be affected by broader and more general disturbances of the body scheme like feeling supernumerary limbs.

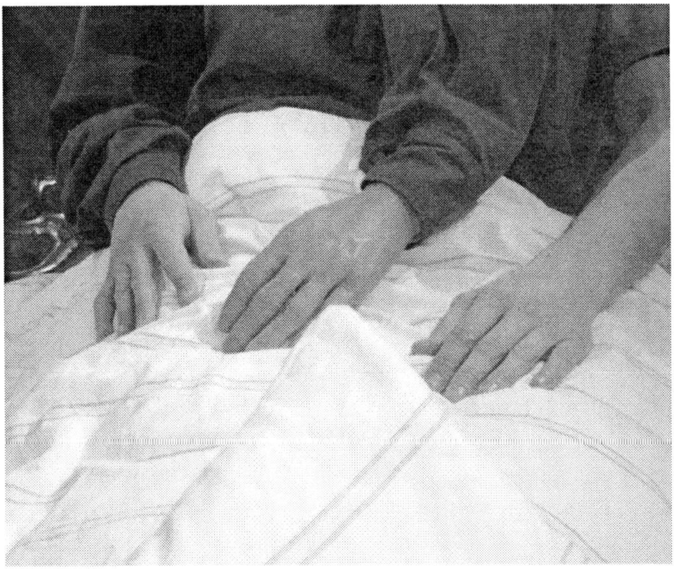

Figure 13. Attachment of the artificial third hand and arm to the body of the participant. The "third" arm was attached between the middle of the body and the left arm.

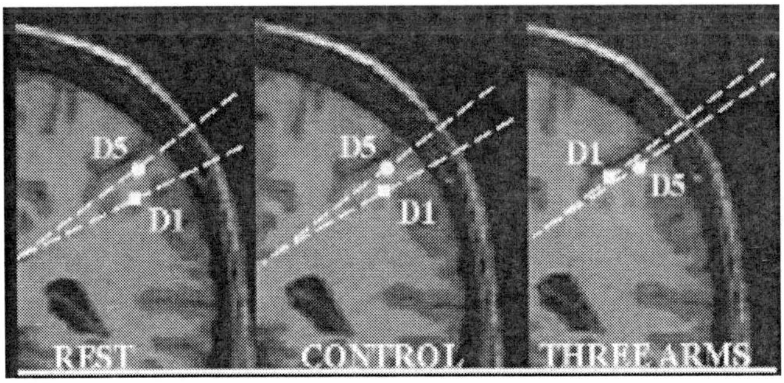

Figure 14. Dipole sources of the SEFs of D1 (squares) and D5 (circles) for one representative subject. Note the differences of the distances for the cortical representations between rest or control condition and illusion condition (three arms), respectively.

It seems remarkable that simply viewing the body “disguised” elicits feelings of a morphed body, associated with modulations in SI topography. Several studies demonstrated that vision can dominate the tactile sense to an extent that subject’s body feelings are modulated or distorted (e.g., Rock and Victor, 1964; Schaefer et al., 2007). Whereas these studies manipulated the visual sense to evoke illusory feelings, other studies changed proprioception (Goodwin et al., 1972) or the tactile sense (Botvinick and Cohen, 1994) to induce similar illusions. However, although the strength of the illusion in the current study seems to be weaker compared with, for example, the rubber-hand illusion (Botvinick and Cohen, 1994), the discussed studies (along with Rock and Victor, 1964) demonstrate that just viewing the body morphed or disguised is sufficient to influence the perception of the body for many subjects. Thus, simply seeing the body as looking different can change the perception and feeling of the body.

We concluded that SI may provide a first dynamic and transient coherent body image by using tactile and also visual information (from other cortical areas via feedback loops, e.g., Rockland and Ojima, 2003). Subsequent cortical processing may then stabilize and enrich this body image with information derived from other modalities. Whereas the body image at this early stage seems to be easily influenced by simple tactile or visual illusions (Chen et al., 2001; Blankenburg et al., 2006; Schaefer et al., 2007, 2008b), later stages of forming the body image might be more influenced by cognitive variables (e.g., in patients with anorexia nervosa).

While many studies describe and examine patients who lost a limb, so far there are only few reports of patients who feel supernumerary phantom limbs. Hari et al., (1998) and McGonigle et al. (2002) report an fMRI case study of patient E.P. with a right frontomesial lesion who sporadically experiences a supernumerary “ghost” arm. Neuromagnetic recordings revealed that activity of the left secondary somatosensory cortex was strongly suppressed during the perception of the ghost arm (Hari et al., 1998). FMRI results showed activation of the supplementary motor area (SMA) when the ghost arm was present (McGonigle et al., 2002). Another case study is reported by Halligan et al. (1993), who describe a patient after a haematoma within the right basal ganglia. This patient reported to feel a third arm, a feeling that lasted for several months. Although this third arm caused distress for the patient and confused him, he had normal cognition and was fully oriented. Similar case studies are reported by Sellal et al. (1996) and Weinstein et al. (1954). However, since the underlying neural mechanisms for feeling supernumerary phantom limbs after brain lesions still seem to be only little understood, it remains unclear if illusions of having a third arm induced by visual manipulations in healthy subjects as reported in the reported study are based on similar neural circuits.

Early experiments already revealed that in an experimentally induced conflict, vision often is strongly dominant. For example, Rock and Victor (1964) used objects whose visual shape differed because of optical distortions from its tactual shape. Subjects had to simultaneously grasp and view the object and were asked to indicate their impressions of it by drawing it or by matching another object to it. The results demonstrated that in this conflict, vision often dominates the tactile sense, even in situations where the observer is not aware of a conflict.

The importance of visual feedback for constructing the body image is well known. Several early studies report that vision also dominates the perception of body parts. For example, Tastevin (1937) showed that people mistook a plastic finger extending beyond a cloth as their own when the latter was concealed several centimeters away. Tastevin (1937) used the term "visual capture" of touch to describe this effect. Further, a later study demonstrated that even when the participants knew they were looking at the experimenter's finger instead of their adjacent occluded fingers, they felt as though the experimenter finger was their own (Welch, 1972).

More recent studies provide further support for this so-called "visual capture" of touch. Pavani et al. (2000) instructed subjects to discriminate the location of vibrotactile stimuli while ignoring distractor lights at various locations. The hands of the subjects were occluded under a table. The results showed that the tactile discriminations were slowed when the distractor light was incongruent with the tactile target rather than congruent, in particular when the light appeared near the stimulated hand. More interestingly, the effect of the distractor lights increased when rubber hands were placed on the table, but only when these rubber hands were spatially (or anatomically) aligned with the participant's own hands. In those conditions, subjects reported the illusion of feeling the touch at the rubber hands.

In a fascinating study, Karin Hägni and colleagues provided further support for the dominance of the visual modality by demonstrating that "visual capture" of touch can arise very easily just by observing and without any further manipulation of vision and touch (Hägni et al., 2008). In this simple experiment, they seated two groups of subjects in front of a monitor watching slow movements of two virtual arms in first-person perspective performing simple goal-directed movements. Whereas one group was instructed to simply observe this scene, the other group was told to imagine that the virtual arms were their own. After about one minute, the virtual arm suddenly was "stabbed" by a knife and began "bleeding." Both groups showed a significant increase in skin conductance. Furthermore, the imagery group showed a significant higher skin conductance than the observation-only group. The authors concluded that even this simple visual imagery was sufficient to at least temporarily incorporate external objects into body image. It has to be stressed that in both conditions, the subjects seemed to have felt the virtual arms. Thus, even without explicitly telling a participant to imagine a robotic arm to be one's own arm, the simple observation of a virtual or robotic arm in first-person perspective seems enough to change the body image. However, it remains unclear what brain regions may be involved in this incorporation of virtual arms, as well as in the other above-mentioned behavioral studies. Nevertheless, based on the results of our studies that we discussed in this chapter, we assume that somatosensory cortices and especially SI plays a key role in creating the here-distorted or "morphed" body image.

But why it is possible to incorporate or "feel" body parts that we can see but do not receive any tactile sensations from? What is the reason for this dominance of the visual sense related to the sense of touch? According to Dawkins (1996) and Ramachandran (1998), tactile sensations are localized directly on the surface where the receptors are actually located. In contrast, visual sensations are "projected" onto the external world. Thus, when light from a tree hits our retinal receptors, we localize the tree externally, not inside our eyeballs. In this sense, vision works like a "remote sensing" device, which liberates ourselves from the requirement of direct contact with the object we are trying to localize. Thus, viewing a virtual arm on a computer screen that suddenly is "stabbed" by a knife or just seeing a third hand attached to our bodies makes us very easily "feel" the touch and body part. As we will see later, the results of these experiments may also be used as new therapeutic approaches for patients with distortions of the body image, for example patients with phantom-limb pain (see chapter 9).

Chapter 7

My Body and Your Body: SI and the Social World

Orlac looks again and again at his hands. What had he done? What had these hands done? Those hands, which were attached to his body but originally belonged to another man. He murdered someone, although he never wanted to do this. It were the hands that did this, it was not really himself, just these strange hands. In the German expressionistic movie *The Hands of Orlac* by Robert Wiene, a pianist has a transplant operation that gives him new hands. Unfortunately, the hands belonged to a murderer, and Orlac suddenly finds himself in a situation in which his new hands commit crimes and start to take over his life. Although today this idea sounds bizarre, we are still fascinated when we hear that not only hands but also even parts of faces have been transplanted. Thus, in contrast to contemporary views, which describe the location of the sense of self somewhere in the brain, we often still seem to think that also body parts somehow represent parts of our selves. Recent experiments that I will discuss in this chapter show us how important it is to know that some body parts belong to our bodies and others do not. Further, these studies also report how easily this basic knowledge can be manipulated, resulting in distorted body schemas. Moreover, the experiments will demonstrate that even SI as a very early stage of cortical processing maintains important functions regarding the difference between the perception of one's own body and bodies of others. Given this capability, a further function of the somatosensory cortices seems to be the perception of social aspects of a situation.

The studies reported above have shown that in contrast to traditional views, SI seems to have a much more complex role than previously assumed. SI is not only prone to influences from motor or premotor areas, even prefrontal areas seem to have an impact on this brain region. Further, SI reflects the perceived body image rather than the actual location of physical stimulation. In addition, recent studies also relate the somatosensory cortices to higher cognitive functions, e.g., the representation of peripersonal space and even social perception, which we will discuss in the following section.

In general, healthy subjects know very well what belongs to their own bodies. However, as discussed above, simple manipulations in multisensory integration can induce profound tactile illusions. Based on these simple manipulations, Botvinick and Cohen (1998) reported an intriguing finding. They instructed participants to watch a rubber hand placed on a table in front of them. Their real right hands were hidden. Now the experimenter touched both, the real right hand as well as the rubber hand, with a small paintbrush. After a few seconds, the participants reported an astonishing feeling: they perceive the touch sensations as arising from the rubber hand, when both the rubber hand and their own real hidden hands were repeatedly tapped in synchrony (Botvinick and Cohen, 1998; Armel and Ramachandran, 2003). Thus, subjects had the feeling as if the rubber hand belonged to their own bodies! This illusion disappeared when a small asynchrony was introduced between the stroking of the rubber and the real hand. The effect of the rubber hand illusion was replicated in many studies (e.g., Makin et al. 2008; Ehrsson et al. 2004; Ehrsson et al. 2005). For example, in a study by Ehrsson et al. (2008), the rubber-hand illusion was used in upper limb amputees to evoke feelings of ownership for the rubber hands replacing their lost hands. This was accomplished by simultaneously touching the stump of the amputees and the fingers of the rubber hands. In another study, Durgin et al. (2007) showed that even touches from a light beam are sufficient to evoke the rubber-hand illusion. The authors reported that touching a rubber hand with a bright beam of light from a laser pointer generated tactile and thermal sensations when the rubber hand was seen as one's own hand.

What are the neural correlates for this manipulation of ownership of an alien body part? Animal data suggest an involvement of the posterior parietal cortex in this projection of sensations to external limbs (Graziano et al., 2000). Further, fMRI data revealed an involvement of the premotor cortex and areas in the PPC when feeling the rubber-hand illusion (Ehrsson et al., 2004, 2005). Interestingly, Peled et al. (2003) found altered somatosensory evoked potentials in schizophrenic patients during the rubber-hand illusion, proposing a role of the somatosensory cortices when subjects report feelings of ownership regarding the rubber hand.

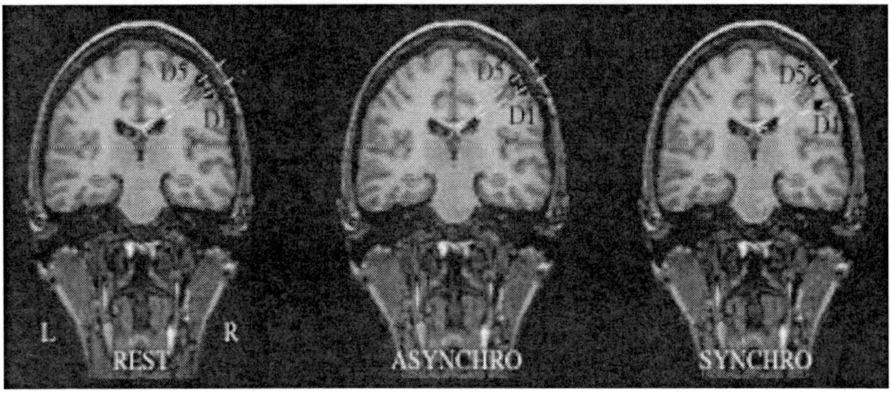

Figure 15. Dipole sources of the SEFs. Note the differences between rest or asynchronous condition (asynchro) and synchronous (synchro) condition.

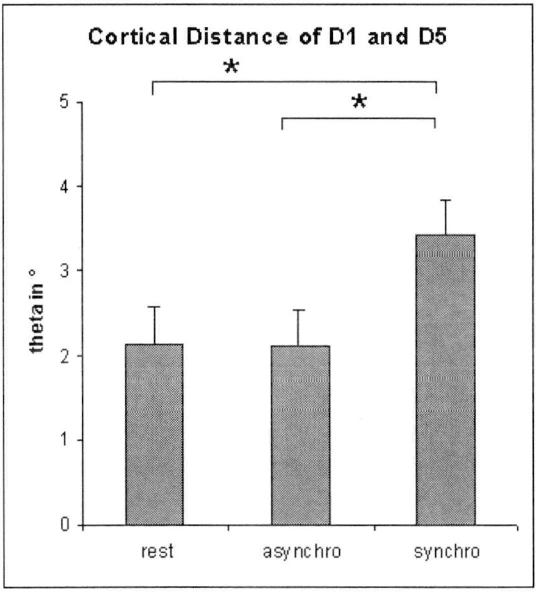

Figure 16. Mean differences (group data) between D1 and D5 dipoles during rest, asynchronous and synchronous condition (D5 always rest state). Asterisks indicate the significant differences between the synchronous (synchro) and asynchronous (asynchro) condition and rest, respectively.

To further test whether the rubber-hand illusion engages SI, we conducted an MEG study (Schaefer et al., 2006b). We recorded neuromagnetic fields while subjects watched a video showing a hand that was stroked by a stick on D1. At the same time, subjects were stimulated on D1, synchronously or asynchronously to the stimulated hand in the video. The video was displayed in the peripersonal space of the subjects. Based on the findings of Botvinick and Cohen (1998), we assumed that during synchronous stimulation, the subjects would experience an illusion of feeling the touch on the hand in the video. We further hypothesized that the cortical representation of D1 would be modulated, suggesting dynamic short-term modulations of cortical maps related to this illusion.

Behavioral results showed that indeed in the synchronous stimulation condition, subjects reported an illusion in which they stated that they felt as if they were being touched on the hands in the video and that they could "feel" the video hand as their own hands. Results of the neuromagnetic source imaging revealed that the cortical representation of D1 changed to a more inferior location during synchronous (the illusion condition) in comparison to asynchronous stimulation and baseline (Figs. 15 and 16). Moreover, this change was significantly positively correlated with the feeling of the touch on the video hand. The more the subjects felt the video hand as their own hands, the more the cortical representation of the real hand was shifting. Thus, the data suggest that somatosensory cortical maps contribute to the experienced illusion in which the subjects seemed to feel the touching of the hand on the video hand. Only if the seen touch was attributed to the body, SI seems to be modulated. Hence, the results demonstrate that viewing touch in peripersonal space can change somatosensory processing in SI when it is believed to occur on the own body, but not when it is believed to be on the body of someone else.

The rubber-hand paradigm, which was originally reported by Botvinick and Cohen in 1998, has drawn much attention in the last years. The basic mechanism has been developed to induce even more astonishing perceptual illusions. For instance, based on an adopted rubber-hand paradigm, Ehrsson (2007) reported a fascinating perceptual illusion in which subjects experience that their "self" is located outside their physical body and that they look at their bodies from the perspective of another person (the so-called out-of-body-experience [OBE], Ehrsson et al., 2007; Lenggenhager et al., 2007). So far, the neural correlates of these illusions remain unclear. We assume that similar neural mechanisms as in the rubber-hand illusion are involved in this kind of illusion. Since the whole body (instead of only parts of it) here is subject to change, it is reasonable to assume additional brain regions involved in this illusion. In further experiments, the group of Ehrsson also reported that it is possible to swap his or her body with that of another person (Petkova and Ehrsson, 2008). They manipulated the visual perspective in combination with the receipt of correlated multisensory information from the body to induce the illusion that another person's body was one's own. Furthermore, by using an analogue paradigm, Petkova and Ehrsson (2008) also demonstrated that one can swap into an artificial body. In a recent study, Petkova and Ehrsson (2009) varied the paradigm again and showed referral of touch and ownership between the hands. Thus, they elicited an illusion where subjects experience "phantom touches" on a right rubber hand when they see it brushed simultaneously with brushes applied to their left hands. The participants reported a duplication and transfer of touch from the left to the right hand, similar to the referral of touch we discussed in patients with phantom sensations subsequent to upper limb amputation (see chapter 2). It remains an open question if and how somatosensory cortices are involved in this kind of illusion.

The results of the study discussed above (Schaefer et al., 2006b) bring up some further questions. To what extent are the somatosensory cortices capable of understanding touch seen on a body? Perhaps the somatosensory cortices already may be activated merely by the *observation* of touch, in the absence of any real touch? In other words, is there something like a mirror neuron system for observed and experienced touch, analogue to the mirror neuron system for action observation?

Let us first briefly discuss the famous theory of a mirror neuron system for observation and execution of actions. The mirror neuron system for action observation has been introduced by Rizzolatti et al. (1996a). Previous animal studies have found so-called mirror neurons in monkey area F5. These neurons discharge with the performance of goal-directed actions and also with observation of another individual performing a similar action (Di Pellegrino et al., 1992; Gallese et al., 1996; Rizzolatti et al., 1996a; Rizzolatti et al., 1996b). These properties of the neurons may build the neural basis for a mechanism that allows matching between visual description of an action and its execution. Thus, a mirror neuron system for action observation is suggested. This mirror neuron system for action observation may be related to action recognition and action understanding. Action understanding means to get an internal description of an action, which might be used for organizing appropriate behavior. According to the mirror theory, this is not based on the visual analysis of different elements of the observed action and subsequent inferences. Rather, this is based on the mapping of visual representation of the observed action onto our motor representation. Hence, we understand others through an internal act that recaptures the sense of their acting (Rizzolatti et al., 2001).

An increasing body of evidence suggests a mirror system in humans similar to that described in the monkey. Imaging studies propose the presence of mirror neurons in several cortical areas, in particular the ventral premotor area, which is the homologue region to the monkey F5 area (Rizzolatti et al., 1996; Grafton et al., 1996; Iacaboni et al., 1999; Buccino et al., 2001; Avikainen et al., 2002). Further, a number of studies suggest an involvement of the primary motor area, which might be activated through premotor areas (Fadiga et al., 1995; Hari et al., 1998; Gangitano et al., 2001).

Several animal studies also found neurons in the parietal cortex, which are responding both to tactile stimulation and to visual stimuli (e.g., Iriki et al., 1996; Graziano et al., 1999). Further, recent evidence suggests that some neurons in the primary somatosensory cortex (SI) are able to code arbitrary visual-tactile associations: Animal studies have shown that neurons in monkey SI may fire both in response to a tactile stimulus and also in response to a visual stimulus previously associated with the tactile stimulus (Zhou et al., 1997). Some of these neurons even showed sustained activity during the visual-tactile delay period, thus suggesting a cross-modal short-term memory (Zhou et al., 2000). This process could involve either a local mechanism within SI, or interactions with other cortical areas (parietal cortex), or a combination of both. The interaction with the parietal cortex may involve bimodal neurons, which are sensitive both for vision and touch. Hence, analogue to the mirror system for action observation, a possible mirror system for observing and receiving touch may exist. This mirror system might be based on the activation of sensory cortical areas, which are linked to areas containing bimodal neurons.

Understanding of the sense of observed touch is an essential ability. Touch can be meant friendly, dangerous, or goal directed. According to the mirror theory, observation of touch might be important for the recognition and understanding of the touch, for getting an internal description, understanding of what happens and to organize appropriate behavior. Thus, a mirror neuron system for tactile observation analogue to action observation could be crucial for fast assessment and evaluation of a situation.

The neuronal correlates of observing tactile stimulation are mainly unknown. In order to determine the pattern of brain activation related to the observation of touch, we conducted an fMRI study, in which subjects watched a video showing a hand that is touched on the index finger by a paintbrush in a repetitive way. In a control condition, the subjects watched again the video hand and the paintbrush, but this time the paintbrush did not touch the hand. Thus, the control condition included the same motion and visual aspects as in the experimental condition. Subjects viewed a touched hand either in an allocentric view or in an egocentric perspective (in the absence of any real touch) (Figure 17). We hypothesized that the observation of the tactile stimulation would lead to an activation of SI, similar to the activation evoked by real stimulation with the paintbrush. This would give an important hint for a mirror system for observed and received touch.

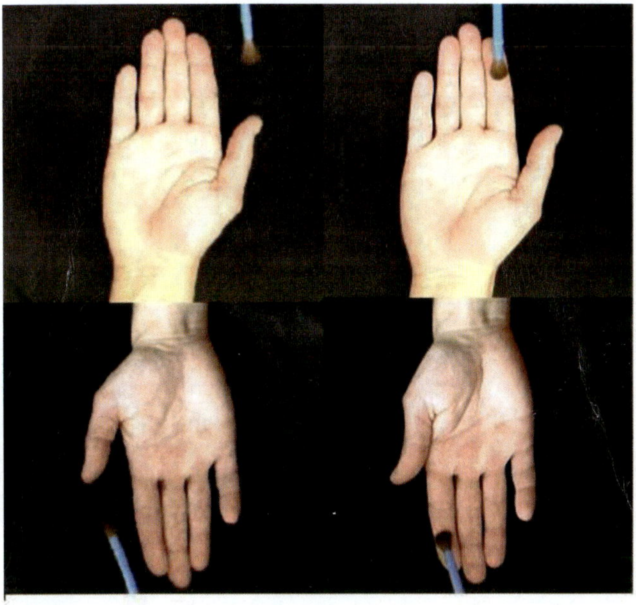

Figure 17. Conditions of the experiment: On the right, the touch-condition; on the left, the non-touch condition. The upper panel depicts the hand in egocentric perspective, the lower in the allocentric perspective.

A mirror neuron system for observed touch may have important implications for rehabilitation of somatosensory impaired patients, for example after stroke. Stroke often affects the somatosensory domain. There are only few rehabilitative treatments that are focused specifically on somatosensory recovery. It would be desirable to develop strategies to enhance sensory performance, especially in forms that do not rely on physical training, because many patients are unable to perform physical training.

The results revealed activation of somatosensory cortices (SI and SII) when observing the hand being touched in egocentric as well as in the allocentric perspective, in the absence of any real touch on the hands (see Figure 18). Thus, a touched hand that we are only watching in a movie is sufficient to evoke an activation of our somatosensory cortices, a region that once was thought to merely reflect physical stimulation on our own body! Based on these results, we concluded that SI seems to be capable of much more than we previously thought in this brain area, even processing touch seen on other's body.

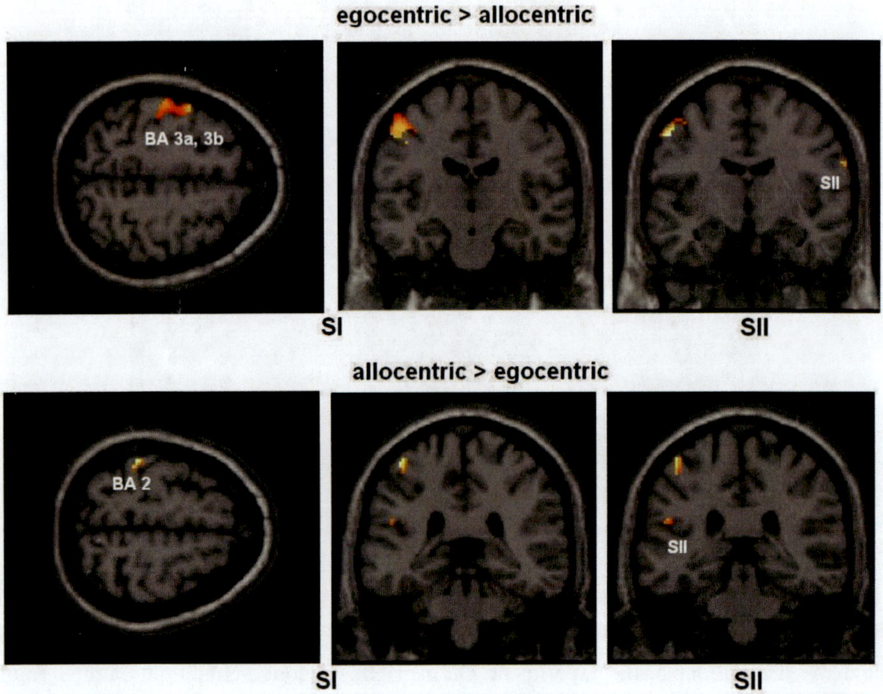

Figure 18. Brain response for observed touch (relative to nontouch) in egocentric perspective compared with neural activations for allocentric perspective, superimposed on the MNI reference brain. Results show significant posterior activation of SI for the allocentric perspective (BA 2) relative to the egocentric perspective (BA 3a, 3b).

Even more fascinating was that the somatosensory cortices seem to be activated differentially depending on the perspective of the observed touch. Whereas the egocentric perspective showed activation in the anterior part of SI (BA 3a, 3b), the allocentric perspective involved significant activation of the posterior part of SI (BA 2) (Figure 15). BA 2 has multimodal receptive fields and connections to the rostral part of the posterior parietal cortex, which, in turn, receives visual input from more caudal parts of the posterior parietal cortex (Iwamura, 1998). Thus, the connectivity between these regions may be related to the activation in BA 2. Viewing touch in an egocentric condition may have induced self-attribution/imagination of being touched on one's own hand, which is different from observing touch on another hand, and which might require less multimodal activation in BA 2. Feeling/imagining being touched oneself may engage a slightly different neural network that requires less multimodal activation in BA 2. Since it is difficult to separate clearly SI in different Brodman areas by using fMRI, these interpretations remain speculative. Nevertheless, results of another recent study support the idea of a functional dissociation in SI. Ebisch et al. (2008) used fMRI to examine whether the tactile mirror mechanism applies to the sight of any touch, irrespective of the intentionality of the observed touching agent. They found a shared neural circuitry for touch in SII and a significant difference between the sight of an intentional touch compared to an accidental touch in left SI/BA 2. The activity in SI/BA 2 was correlated with the degree of intentionality of the seen touch. The authors concluded that this activity in SI may reflect a human tendency to resonate more with an intentional touch agent than with an accidentally touched object. In our study, when touch was viewed in an allocentric viewing perspective, brain activation was observed in SI/BA 2. These results are consistent with the findings reported in Ebisch et al. (2008) and further suggest that SI/BA 2 may differentially respond to non-egocentric body contact.

Taken together, SI seems to be differentially engaged depending on whether observed touch is attributed to one's own body or to someone else. Moreover, different parts of SI seem to provide different functions regarding the differentiation of self and others and also depending on the perceived intentionality of the seen touch. Hence, we conclude that SI seems to be involved when perceiving social situations.

The results of this study showing activation of somatosensory areas when observing touch are discussed in terms of a possible mirror neuron system for observed and experienced touch (e.g., Keysers et al., 2004; Blakemore et al., 2005). The results are consistent with previous findings regarding activation of SI and SII when observing a touched face (e.g., Blakemore et al., 2005), providing further support for a potential mirror system of sensory observation. Whereas the mirror neuron system of action observation seems to be crucial for the understanding and imitation of actions (Rizzolatti et al., 2001) and for the understanding of intentions (Iacoboni et al., 2005; Iacoboni and Dapretto, 2006), a mirror neuron system for observation of touch may be important for the recognition and understanding of touch. This may be crucial to form an internal representation of a somatosensory event and to estimate consequences necessary for action preparation. Thus, a mirror neuron system for tactile observation analogous to action observation may exist that might be necessary for rapid assessment and evaluation of how other people may feel or a situation that may be consequential to the observer.

Keysers et al., as well as Ebisch et al., demonstrated somatosensory activations when touch is observed, irrespective of what is being touched, animate subjects or inanimate objects. In contrast, our study examined only touch of an animate object (a human hand). It remains an issue whether the activation of SI/BA 2 would be similar, irrespective of the animacy of the observed object. In contrast to the mirror system for actions, it is possible that the mirror system for touch is not limited to a social context, which would be consistent with previous results (Keysers et al., 2004; Ebisch et al., 2008).

A recent fMRI study also looked for brain activations when a hand is depicted in ego- vs. allocentric perspectives, but here the authors focused on the mirror neuron theory for *action* observation (Shmuelof and Zohary, 2008). In their experiment, the authors showed hands that manipulated a cube, or they asked the subjects to make self-performed actions. Shmuelof and Zohary found a mirror-image representation of others' actions (allocentric view) in the anterior parietal cortex. Viewing egocentric-based actions revealed greater fMRI activation in the contralateral hemisphere. Based on these results, the authors suggest an automatic action–simulation system in the parietal cortex. Thus, the results of Shmuelof and Zohary (2008) report results for the mirror neuron system for action observation convergent with the mirror system for observation of touch regarding its sensitivity on the perceived perspective of the seen body part.

Chapter 8

DR. STRANGELOVE AND THE EVIL HAND

When W.H. wakes up in the morning, he has to be very careful with his left hand. Don't wake it up to roughly! W.H. gently touches his left hand, and it slowly moves upward beneath the blanket, resting in this position. It is a good day today, and the hand is not hostile to W.H., who is the owner of the hand. It was not always like that. On bad days, the hand was doing what it wanted, causing many problems for W.H. For example, W.H. wanted to pick up the phone with his right and healthy hand, but the left alien hand also grasped for the phone and tried to hang up. W.H. remembers days in which both hands almost were fighting against each other. In some situations, the left and alien hand was doing things that were not only strange for W.H. but also very inconvenient. For instance, the left hand covered his face and rested upon it with great strength. W.H. had to use his healthy hand to force the alien hand move away from his face. In fact, there were situations in which the alien hand was really aggressive and dangerous: The hand moved up to his neck, grasped and throttled it, while W.H. desperately tried to use his healthy hand to restrain the alien hand.

W.H. is a patient with a bizarre disorder called alien-hand or alien-limb syndrome. This striking phenomenon has fascinated not only scientists but also philosophers and artists. Perhaps the most prominent example is that of Dr. Strangelove, the main character of Stanley Kubrick's movie *Dr. Strangelove or How I Learned to Stop Worrying and Love the Bomb.* He is described as erratic and shows this bizarre movement disorder. His right hand seems to be out of control and having a will of its own. Sometimes it grasps his throat, and Dr. Strangelove must try to restrain this limb with his other hand, just the way W.H. told us. There are also times when this alien hand raises into a Nazi salute, making the figure of Dr. Strangelove even more bizarre. Although this character is, of course, fictional, the very rare symptom of an alien hand can occur in neurological disease. Patients experience the alien limb as being controlled by an external agent and describe it in the third person.

What has happened in patients with this kind of movement disorder? Although there are some reports on alien hands, most of them are descriptive or anecdotal. The alien-hand syndrome most commonly occurs after lesions in the frontal lobes and in the corpus callosum (Gazzaniga et al., 1970). In the year 1908, in one of the first reports on alien hands, Goldstein described a patient who developed left alien-hand behavior after a right anterior cerebral artery infection: "On one occasion, the hand grabbed her own neck and tried to throttle her, and could only be pulled off by force. Similarly, it tore off the bedcovers against the patient's will. ...She soon is complaining about her hand: 'I myself can do nothing with it; if I'm having a drink and it gets hold of the glass, it won't let go and spills [the drink] out. Then I hit it and say: "Behave yourself, hand." (smiling) I suppose there must be an evil spirit in it.'"

The alien-hand syndrome is also encountered with strokes in the posterior brain, which is then called posterior alien-hand syndrome. Further, an alien hand sometimes is reported in patients with corticobasal degeneration, a progressive neurodegenerative condition in which there is both cortical and basal ganglia dysfunction. W.H., who was a patient in our clinic and whose story introduced this chapter, was diagnosed with this disease.

The different underlying neural diseases causing the alien hand are related to different clinical signs. Thus, in patients with corticobasal degeneration, there are different movement abnormalities regarding the alien limb compared with patients with lesions in the frontal lobe or corpus callosum. For example, perseverative movements in patients with corticobasal degeneration are less common. What neural systems are disabled in patients with corticobasal degeneration, the diagnosis W.H. received in our clinic? Although the exact location of areas with neural degeneration is difficult to specify, regions in posterior frontal lobe as well as in anterior parietal lobe seem to be most severely affected.

Since the alien-hand syndrome is a rare neurological disorder, so far, only few studies used experimental approaches to examine its underlying neural network. In an fMRI study, Assal et al. (2007) examined a patient with alien-hand syndrome after right parietal lesion. The results revealed that movements of the alien hand engaged a selective activation of contralateral M1. The authors suggested that this region might be released from conscious control. In contrast, voluntary movements involved a network of active regions, including not only M1 but also premotor cortex and left inferior frontal gyrus. However, since Assal et al. (2007) only reported a single case study, it remains unclear if the results can be generalized. Moreover, we do not know if alien-hand syndromes based on other lesions or neurodegenerative disorders rely on a similar disconnection from M1 to other cortical regions normally involved in movement-planning behavior.

To learn more about the bizarre phenomena, we asked W.H. to participate in a series of different behavioral experiments. Perhaps the most fascinating behavioral study was the rubber-hand experiment. If the left hand became (at least partly) out of control for W.H., would the presentation of a rubber hand stroked synchronously with his real (but alien) hand elicit a much stronger rubber-hand illusion than his healthy hand or as in other subjects? For instance, Peled et al. (2003) used the rubber-hand paradigm to demonstrate that schizophrenic patients are much more prone to the illusion than a control group. Moreover, Peled et al. (2003) were also able to demonstrate that those patients not only felt the illusion more strongly and more vividly, they also showed that these changes were associated with changes even in the somatosensory cortices. In the light of those results, would W.H. also feel the alien rubber hand stronger and more vividly? In other words, in a situation where the body already owns an alien body part, would it be easier for this person to integrate other alien body parts, for example, a rubber hand placed in front of him? Or, in contrast, would it be much more difficult because the body still struggles with an alien body part? The background of this question is the assumption that both phenomena may at least in part rely on the same neural mechanisms. This is reasonable since we know that the rubber-hand illusion is associated with activations in the premotor cortex as well as with areas in the parietal lobe (and in particular also with the somatosensory cortices, see previous chapter). Similar brain areas in the various diseases causing the alien-hand syndrome are also discussed, in particular for patients with corticobasal degeneration. So, does the experimental induction of the ownership of an alien hand interact with the lack of ownership feeling of W.H.'s real alien hand?

To investigate this question, we invited W.H. to participate in the classic rubber-hand experiment (Botvinick and Cohen, 1998). We placed a rubber hand in front of him on a table and asked him to put his left alien hand below this table. Then, we started to brush both the rubber hand and the real hand below the table in a synchronous way, which usually elicits the strong feeling of ownership for this rubber hand. However, the manipulation failed to evoke the well-known rubber-hand illusion in W.H. We concluded that the rubber-hand illusion does not work for subjects with the alien-hand syndrome (at least in the case of W.H.).

Nevertheless, this was only true for his left alien hand. When we asked W.H. to put his healthy right hand below the table, he stated that he had the strong feeling that the rubber hand is his own hand. Hence, for his healthy hand, the illusion seemed to work. However, when we further asked W.H. to point at the position of his hidden real hand with his other hand, W.H. showed an astonishing behavior. In general, healthy subjects mislocalize their real hidden hand in the direction of the rubber hand. This drift is known to be strongly associated with the strength of the rubber-hand illusion. Thus, the more the participants feel the illusion, the more this drift occurs (Botvinick and Cohen, 1998). In the case of W.H., this drift was different. He pointed at a position in the opposite direction, meaning away from the rubber hand. We observed this surprising behavior also mildly in the asynchronous condition.

What may be the reason for this drift in the opposite direction? When subjects are asked to point at their real hidden hands underneath the table, they do this with their other hands. In W.H., the rubber-hand illusion worked only for his healthy right hand. However, when he had to point to the position of the hand under the table, of course he used his left hand, which is his alien hand. We believe that in this pointing task, both hands were in a situation of intermanual conflict. We described those situations above (see also the bimanual coordination experiment in chapter 3). A famous example is when the phone rings and the healthy hand tries to pick up the phone but the alien hand acts in a contradictory way and tries to hang up. A similar situation seems to occur in the rubber-hand paradigm when we asked W.H. to use his alien hand to point to the hidden position of his healthy hand. This behavior seems remarkable if we consider that the healthy hand was not acting at all; it received just passive touch in the experiment finished immediately before. Hence, the situation can be described as an intermanual body image conflict rather than an intermanual acting conflict.

Previous neuroimaging studies revealed that the rubber-hand illusion is associated with an activation of the ventral premotor cortex (Ehrsson et al., 2004), an area that is known to be related to multisensory processing. Further, areas in the posterior parietal cortex (Ehrsson et al., 2004) and in SI (Schaefer et al., 2006b) seem to be involved. Does the lack of the rubber-hand illusion for W.H.'s alien hand refer to a neural distortion of multisensory areas, for instance, the ventral premotor cortex or areas in posterior parietal cortex? To test if activity in multisensory brain areas really reflects the feeling of body ownership in the rubber hand illusion, Ehrsson et al. (2005) suggested an altered rubber-hand paradigm. Here, the experimenter moved the blindfolded participant's left index finger so that it touched the fake hand. Simultaneously to this manipulation, he touched the participant's real right hand. Ehrsson et al. (2005) reported that this manipulation yielded an illusion that one was touching one's own hand and that this impression was associated with activity in ventral premotor areas and intraparietal cortices, suggesting that brain activity here reflects the detection of congruent multisensory signals from one's own body, rather than simply visual representations of the rubber hand in the peripersonal space due to the dominant role of vision. In order to examine if those brain areas may be involved in the lack of the rubber-hand illusion for W.H.'s alien hand, we adopted the paradigm of Ehrsson et al. (2005). We asked W.H. to participate in a second experiment, where we tried to replicate the altered rubber-hand illusion paradigm Ehrsson et al. (2005) has introduced. If those multisensory areas are responsible for the lack of feeling the rubber-hand illusion, then this altered paradigm of Ehrsson et al. (2005) should also fail to show any effects.

Surprisingly, W.H. here reported to feel the illusion even with his alien hand! When we tested the healthy hand, he stated feeling a similar illusion. Moreover, we were also astonished to observe what happened when W.H., this time, was asked to point to the position of his real hidden (healthy) hand. Again, W.H. needed to use his alien hand to perform this part of the task. In fact, now W.H. showed a drift to the expected direction of the rubber hand (instead in the opposite direction, as in the previous experiment)! Thus, we concluded that the dominant role of vision in the first rubber-hand experiment seemed to cause the intermanual conflict of the hands, resulting in an unexpected drift away from the rubber hand in the first study and in the lack of any illusions for his left alien hand. Hence, it seems that more than a just disconnection of the primary motor area (M1) causes the alien hand syndrome—at least in our patient W.H. In contrast, several brain areas seem to be involved, probably linked to multisensory processing and in particular also in processing visual information about what is happening in the peripersonal space.

In the previous chapter, we have seen that we can induce phantoms in normal individuals just by manipulating multisensory integration processes. Further, an increasing body of evidence demonstrated that the somatosensory cortices and especially the functional topography in SI seem to be involved in this kind of illusion. Based on these results, we hypothesized that at least for some diseases that cause the alien-hand syndrome, distortions in the functional topography in SI might play an important role. In order to prove this hypothesis, we tried to examine the functional topography of SI in patient W.H. Given that SI represents the perceived rather than the physical image of the body, it seems likely that the cortical representations of his alien hand are different compared to his healthy limb.

To test the hypothesis that SI may be altered in W.H., we mapped the somatosensory cortices by using neuromagnetic source imaging. The results revealed a comparable somatosensory homunculus for the healthy hand as well as for the alien hand. However, to detect small modulations in the topography of SI, we need to have at least a small sample of those patients. Currently, we are working to define this group, which will enable us to compare the cortical representation of the alien hand with that of the healthy hand, as well as with a control group. The forthcoming results will tell us if and how the somatosensory cortices in patients with alien-hand syndromes are distorted and how this is related to the intriguing phenomena we can observe in those patients.

Chapter 9

USING THE DYNAMIC FACET OF THE BODY IMAGE FOR NEUROREHABILITATION

The studies discussed above have shown that the functional topography in SI seems to vary dynamically and to represent the perceived rather than the physical information of what happen on the skin of the body. The question arises, if and how these results may open the way for new therapeutic approaches, e.g., for patients suffering from phantom-limb pain or from sensory loss in their hands, which is a frequent consequence after stroke. This chapter will review only some new ideas that may once find their way into practical neurorehabiliation.

At present, first approaches trying to use manipulations in multisensory integration to evoke beneficial effects in neurehabiliation are tested. Serino et al. (2007) investigated whether the effect that viewing the body improves tactile acuity (visuo-tactile enhancement, Kennett et al., 2001) might be useful in improving somatosensory deficits of brain-damaged patients (see also chapter 5). Ten of these patients who suffered from a reduced somatosensory sensitivity participated in two-point-discrimination tasks while they had to look at their stimulated forearm, at a neutral object (control condition), and at a rubber hand (control condition). The authors reported an amelioration of the performance in the viewing arm condition, as expected. Thus, the authors suggested that a therapeutic approach based on this visuo-tactile enhancement might be effective in ameliorating somatosensory deficits based, for example, on stroke. However, although it is known that the effects of visuo-tactile enhancement can last up to several minutes (Taylor-Clarke et al., 2002; Ro et al., 2004), it remains unclear how one could stabilize these improvements over a longer time range. Thus, follow-up studies are needed to assess the stability of these training effects.

This argument also dampens enthusiasm about, in principle, encouraging results from another approach. Manipulating the interaction between vision and touch, Ramachandran used a simple and intriguing technique to reduce phantom-limb pain (similar, Sathian et al., 2000; Hunter et al., 2003). According to Ramachandran, the problem of the phantom arm is that it is a learned paralysis. Thus, these patients had to unlearn this paralysis. The patient needs to receive a visual feedback message that his arm is, indeed, moving correctly. Unfortunately, this is not possible since the patient has no arm anymore. To solve this problem, Ramachandran invented a simple box called "virtual reality box." This box enabled the patient to perceive real movement in a non-existent arm, because it had a vertical mirror inside. The front of the simple box had two holes in it, through which the patient inserts his good arm and his "phantom arm." Ramachandran now asked the patient to look into the mirror, which created the illusion of having two hands, because the patient is seeing also the mirror reflection of the intact hand. If the patient now tried to move both arms symmetrically, his brain receives positive visual feedback that his phantom arm is moving correctly, and the patient gets the illusion that his amputated hand has returned. Ramachandran and colleagues used this "virtual reality box" on several patients with phantom-limb pain and reported encouraging results (Ramachandran and Hirstein, 1998). More in detail, they reported that in six of ten patients, the phantom hand was perceived to move in the mirror. Four patients felt no effect on the phantom arm. Further, in four of five patients, who felt involuntary painful "clenching spasms" in the phantom hand, the mirror box relieved the spasms. Moreover, Ramachandran and Hirstein also reported that training with this mirror box (ten minutes per day over three weeks) led to a permanent disappearance of the phantom arm in one patient (or, in the words of Ramachandran and Hirstein, in a successful "amputation" of the phantom limb). However, as the authors stressed themselves, these results have to be followed by better controlled clinical trials to assess the impact of this "virtual reality box."

The "virtual reality box" has been shown to induce vivid kinesthetic sensations of movements in amputees. Altschuler et al. (1999) could demonstrate that this approach of a mirror therapy can also be used for rehabilitation of hemiparesis after stroke, giving the patients the visual impression that their affected arms are moving normally. Altschuler et al. (1999) reported results from nine patients at least six months post-stroke who participated in training with the "virtual reality box" over four weeks, for 15 minutes two times per day. The authors reported that all subjects liked to use the "virtual reality box." More important, the authors found that significantly more patients improved on mirror than on control. The authors conclude that mirror therapy may be beneficial for at least some patients with hemiparesis following stroke.

Although all these studies report interesting results, clinical trials including a larger sample of patients are necessary to assess the validity of the results. Furthermore, imaging data are needed to understand why and how, for instance, the mirror therapy works. So far, it remains unclear what neural structures are involved when manipulations of multisensory integration result in beneficial effects for those patients. It would be desirable to show that certain brain areas are associated with the reported relief of pain or improved skills, as, for example, was shown in the case of sensory training for phantom-limb pain patients (Flor et al., 2001, see above in chapter 2).

Chapter 10

CONCLUSION: CONSEQUENCES FOR THE IMAGE OF OUR SELF

The famous physicist Stephen Hawking once was asked about the reasons for his decision to become a researcher on astronomy and theoretical physics. He answered that he thought that one could either examine the very small things, meaning doing research on atomic physics, or one could investigate the really big and large things, pointing to astronomical research. As we all know, Hawking decided for the latter. However, Hawking missed a third possibility: To look at the observer itself, meaning engaging in neuroscience, and thus investigating the self who is observing both, the space and the atomic structure of the elements. So, given that neuroscientists now have been working for quite a long time, what did we find out, and what is the conclusion we can draw out of the research regarding the image of our self? And, in particular, considering the topic of this book, what is the conclusion for the relationship between body and mind?

Since the early observations of Head and Holmes (1911), it has been well known that there is a stable mental construct of the body or a unitary corporeal self that endures in space and in time. The somatosensory cortices have an important role in maintaining this corporeal self. The above-discussed studies have demonstrated that the functions of SI are much more complex than previously thought. Thus, SI seems to be influenced by higher order cortical sites like prefrontal areas, by tactile illusions or simple masquerades of the body, by manipulations of the visible size of body parts, and also even by social perceptions. The mental construct of the body is supposed to be based on a network of different brain areas, but research discussed above suggests that a corporeal self at a very early stage of sensory processing seems to be established.

Later stages in forming body image might be more influenced by cognitive variables (with probably other distortions of the body image).

This new understanding of the function of SI may encourage approaches that try to use the dynamic facet of this body image as a tool in rehabilitation. For example, recent studies demonstrated that the manipulation of visual feedback can be used to successfully influence phantom sensations in amputees. Studies using the virtual reality box (or mirror-box), which utilizes visual feedback (the mirror image of the intact hand) to pretend the physical occurrence of the phantom limb, report intriguing results, as we have seen in the previous chapter (Ramachandran and Rogers-Ramachandran, 1996; Hunter et al., 2003). Future approaches may also include other patients with distorted body images, e.g., with anorexia nervosa.

However, the major conclusion of the presented results is more fundamental. These studies show that at a very early stage in cortical processing complex, perceptions are being processed in SI, which probably even include social aspects. When SI is capable of perceiving social information, it also needs to maintain a sense of self. This is also warranted by the fact that touch is always twofold: When we feel touch, we receive information at the same time about the external object touching our skin as well as about our body itself. Thus, in contrast to traditional views, central aspects of our self are not only based on frontal brain regions, but also on areas previously thought to be important for more basic processing, the somatosensory cortices. We conclude that our self seems to be based on a very broad network of brain regions, including possibly even the primary processing areas.

But the question regarding the image of our self can also be answered by the way the brain is working. One of the key issues in this book was the suggestion that SI does not simply represent the physical world rather than a world that already has been interpreted or biased. SI seems to actively *perceive* information rather than just simply reflect upon it. Thus, the *meaning* of touch that happens on the body is crucial for coding it in the somatosensory homunculus.

Although we have concentrated on the tactile dimension, similar results have been reported regarding other modalities, e.g., vision or the auditory domain. An example for the auditory domain comes from studies trying to understand tinnitus. Patients having this disease hear tones that normally are physically not present. A neuromagnetic study has revealed that tinnitus patients have distortions in the primary acoustic cortex (AI), which are similar to the cortical reorganization we have known in patients with phantom-limb pain (Mühlnickel et al., 1998). The auditory cortex AI is similarly topographically organized as the homunculus in SI (or MI), locating cortical representations of different frequencies in a tonotopic map. Using MEG, Mühlnickel et al. (1998) determined whether the tonotopy in auditory cortex of tinnitus patients diverges from normative functional organization. Ten tinnitus subjects and a control group were exposed to four sets of tones while neuromagnetic recordings were obtained from both hemispheres. The authors reported a shift of the cortical representation of the tinnitus frequency into an area adjacent to the expected tonotopic location. Moreover, they found a correlation with the subjective ratings of the strengths of the tinnitus and the amount of cortical reorganization (r = . 82). Mühlnickel et al. (1998) concluded that tinnitus seems to be related to plastic changes in the auditory cortex. Further, they compared their results with that of the cortical reorganization in phantom-limb pain patients. Since in both cases alterations or shifts in the primary processing area associated with the disease have been observed, the authors suggest that tinnitus may be an auditory phantom phenomenon.

Further, there are hints that the tonotopic map in AI, similar to SI in the tactile modality, represents the perceived rather than the physical auditory information. Evidence comes from a study with paranoid schizophrenic patients (Dierks et al., 1999). Using fMRI, the authors could demonstrate that auditory hallucinations were associated with an increase of the blood oxygen level-dependent (BOLD) signal in Heschl's gyrus. Thus, the results provide evidence of the involvement of primary auditory areas in auditory verbal hallucinations. These results may also explain why hallucinations are experienced as entirely real (in contrast to auditory imagery or inner speech).

In sum, it seems reasonable to hypothesize that in all primary cortical areas, information of the outer world is not "mechanically" represented. In contrast, it seems that even in very early stages of sensory processing, information always is *perceived* rather than simply physically depicted or reflected. Thus, information is selected and biased even at first cortical processing sites. As a result, one might say that the brain at its "gates" is more "intelligent" than previously thought.

This new look at the brain is in contradiction to traditional views. The classical understanding is that the brain is organized hierarchically and modularly. Thus, this traditional view subdivides the brain into different sections according to the different modalities, e.g., somatosensory cortex, visual cortex, etc. The primary areas of this differentiation have been understood to be unimodal and to depict physical stimuli in a mechanical way. Do the results force us to completely rethink this classic view of our brain? I do not think so. Numerous studies based on imaging, neuropsychological, or animal data have confirmed that the brain is working in general hierarchically and that the first processing areas like V1 or SI are working predominantly unimodally. Nevertheless, the studies we have discussed in this book made clear that this organization of the brain is not absolute, showing, for example, that previously unimodal areas are affected by multimodal processing. Thus, on the one hand, I think that the brain is organized in hierarchies and also in modality specific processing areas, but on the other hand, we should keep in mind that the brain also works partly multimodally, even in primary processing areas and that it also works in a top-down manner in order to achieve and maintain a coherent view of the world, which perhaps might be the main goal of perception.

The last argument also stresses that these topics are not solely a subject of physiology but belong to psychological and philosophical disciplines as well. One prominent example is the work of the French philosopher Maurice Merleau-Ponty, who we already mentioned in the introduction of this book. A major goal of his work was to understand how we perceive our own and another's bodies. Merleau-Ponty argues that one's own body is not only a thing or an object that we can study in science, but also a condition of the perceptual openness to the world. He recognizes an intentionality of the body as well as a corporeity of consciousness, thereby putting himself in opposion of dualistic positions of mind and body suggested mainly by René Descartes (Merleau-Ponty, 1945).

It is astonishing to see that this phenomenological view of perception and the body is in line with recent studies on body perception, as we have discussed them in the chapters before. When early stages of tactile processing are prone to what happens in the peripersonal space, to seen (and only illusionary felt!) body parts, to the perspective of the displayed body parts, and also to new body parts connected with our own bodies, the idea of a corporeity of consciousness as much as an intentionality of the body may explain these phenomena.

But what does Merleau-Ponty mean when he speaks about the intentionality of the body? Does he really mean that the body is doing little things on its own? He argues that insofar "as I have hands, feet; a body, I sustain around me intentions which are not dependent on my decisions and which affect my surroundings in a way that I do not choose" (1945). In this view, Merleau-Ponty also touches the work of other famous phenomonlogical philosophers, namely Edmund Husserl and Martin Heidegger. The last one developed these thoughts further to a coherent new and radical theory of "being in the world" (the German term: "In-der-Welt-sein") (Heidegger, 1927). Taken together, the phenomenological tradition of philosophy offers theories that may be help to explain puzzling phenomena in cognitive neuroscience. However, a disadvantage may be that, so far, both disciplines are working mainly separatly and were developed on their own. Thus, it seems very difficult to work in both worlds trying to converge the results in a coherent theory. As a consequence, today we do not have many convincing theories including philosophical aspects as well as neuroscientific approaches.

This book tried to demonstrate that the percpetion of the body and its representation in the brain is not fixed but dynamic and flexible, explained better by phenomenological theories than machine-like metaphors of rigid representation of body parts. But why does the brain show such a variety and flexibility in its organization? The reason for that is probably that in this way, it tries to maximize its ability to learn and to adapt to different environmental situations, which always can rapidly change. If the brain is also able to adapt to the extremely fast-changing requirements of our modern world (meaning control of emotions, working in virtual environments, or encountering the problem of eating the wrong and too much food instead of too little), remains an open question. So far, we have to say that our brain is doing a great job.

ACKNOWLEDGMENTS

MS was supported by grants of the Deutsche Forschungsgemeinschaft.

REFERENCES

Altschuler, E.L., Wisdom, S.B., Stone, L., Foster, C., Galasko, D., Llewellyn, D.M., Ramachandran, V.S., 1999. Rehabilitation of hemiparesis after stroke with a mirror. *Lancet* 353, 2035-2036.

Anderson, J.R., Douglas, S., 2002. Tower of Hanoi: evidence for the cost of goal retrieval. *J. Exp. Psychol. Learn. Mem. Cogn.* 27, 1331-1346.

Armel, K.C., Ramachandran, V.S., 2003. Projecting sensations to external objects. Evidence from skin conductance response. *Proced. Roy. Soc. Biol. Sci.* 270, 1499-1506

Assal F, Schwartz S, Vuilleumier P., 2007. Moving with or without will: functional neural correlates of alien hand syndrome. *Ann. Neurol.* 62, 301-306.

Avikainen, S., Forss, N., Hari, N., 2002. Modulated activation of human SI and SII cortices during observation of hand actions. *Neuroimage* 15, 640-646.

Blakemore, S.-J., Bristow, D., Bird, G., Frith, C., Ward, J., 2005. Somatosensory activations during the observation of touch and a case of vision-touch synaesthesia. *Brain* 128, 1571-1583.

Blankenburg, F., Ruff, C.C., Deichmann, R., Rees, G., Driver, J., 2006. The cutaneous rabbit illusion affects human primary sensory cortex somatotopically. *PloS. Biol.* 4, e69.

Botvinick, M., Cohen, J., 1998. Rubber hand "feel" touch that eyes can see. *Nature* 391, 756.

Braun, C., Schweizer, R., Elbert, T., Birbaumer, N., Taub, E., 2000. Differential activation in somatosensory cortex for different discrimination tasks. *J. Neurosci.* 20, 446-450.

Braun, C., Heinz, U., Schweizer, R., Wiech, K., Birbaumer, N., Topka, H., 2001. Dynamic organization of the somatosensory cortex induced by motor activity. *Brain* 124, 2259-2267.

Braun, C., Haug, M., Wiech, K., Birbaumer, N., Elbert, T., Roberts, L., 2002. Functional organization of primary somatosensory cortex depends on the focus of attention. *Neuroimage* 17, 1451-1458.

Buccino, G.., Binkofski, F.., Fink, G.R., Fadiga, L., Fogassi, L., Gallese, V., Seitz, R.J., Zilles K., Rizzolatti, G., Freund H.J., 2001. Action observation activates premotor and parietal areas in a somatotopic manner: an fMRI study. *Eur. J. Neuroscience* 13, 400-404.

Buchner, H., Kauert, C., Rademacher, I., 1995. Short-term changes of finger representation at the somatosensory cortex in humans. *Neurosci. Lett.* 198, 57-59.

Celnik, P., Webster, B., Glasser, D.M., Cohen, L.G., 2008. Effects of action observation on physical training after stroke. *Stroke* 39, 1814-1820.

Celnik, P., Stefan, K., Hummel, F., Duque, J., Classen, J., Cohen, L.G., 2006. Encoding a motor memory in the older adult by action observation. *Neuroimage* 29, 677-684.

Chapman, C.E., Jiang, W., Lamarre, Y., 1988. Modulation of lemniscal input during conditioned arm movements in the monkey. *Exp. Brain Res.* 72, 316-334.

Chen, L.M., Friedman, R.M., Roe, A.W., 2003. Optical imaging of a tactile illusion in area 3b of the primary somatosensory cortex. *Science* 302, 881-885.

Dawkins, R., 1996. Climbing Mount Improbable. New York: Norton; 1996.

Dierks, T., Linden, D.E., Jandl, M., Formisano, E., Goebel, R., Lanfermann, H., Singer, W., 1999. Activation of Heschl's gyrus during auditory hallucinations. *Neuron* 22, 615-621.

Di Pellegrino, G., Fadiga, L., Fogassi, L., Gallese, V., Rizzolatti, G., 1992. Understanding motor events: a neurophysiological study. *Exp. Brain Res.* 91, 176-180.

Di Pellegrino, G., Ladavas, E., Farne, A. 1997. Seeing where your hands are. *Nature* 388, 730.

Driver, J., Spence, C., 2000. Multisensory perception: beyond modularity and convergence. *Curr. Biol.* 10, 731-735.

Durgin, F.H., Evans, L., Dunphy, N., Klostermann, S., Simmons, K., 2007. Rubber hands feel the touch of light. *Psychol. Sci.* 18, 152-157.

Ebisch, S.J., Perruci, M.G., Ferretti, A., Del Gratta, C., Romani, G.L., Gallese, V., 2008. The sense of touch: Embodied simulation in a visuo-tactile mirroring mechanism for observed animate or inanimate touch. *J. Cogn. Neuroci*. 20, 1-13.

Ehrsson, H.H., Spence, C., Passingham, R.E., 2004. That's my hand! Activity in premotor cortex reflects feeling of ownership of a limb. *Science* 305, 875-877.

Ehrsson, H.H., Holmes, N.P. Passingham, R.E., 2005. Touching a rubber hand: feeling of body ownership is associated with activity in multisensory brain areas. *J. Neurosci.* 9, 10564-10573.

Ehrsson, H.H., Rosen, B., Stockselius, A., Ragnoe, Ch., Koehler, P., Lundborg, G., 2008. Upper limb amputees can be induced to experience a rubber hand as their own. *Brain* 131, 3443-3452.

Ehrsson, H.H., 2007. The experimental induction of out-of-body experiences. *Science* 317, 1048.

Elbert, T., Pantev, C., Wienbruch, C., Rockstroh, B., Taub, E., 1995. Increased cortical representation of the fingers of the left hand in string players. *Science* 270, 305-307.

Fadiga, L., Fogassi, L., Pavesi, G., Rizzolatti, G., 1995. Motor facilitation during action observation: a magnetic stimulation study. *J. Neurophysiol.* 73, 2608-2611.

Fink, G., Marshall, J.C., Halligan, P.W, Frith, C.D., Driver, J., Frackowiak, R.S., Dolan, R.J., 1999. The neural consequences of conflict between intention and the senses. *Brain* 122, 497-512.

Flor, H., Elbert, T., Knecht, S., Wienbruch, C., Pantev, C., Birbaumer, N., Larbig, W., Taub, E., 1995. Phantom-limb pain as a perceptual correlate of massive reorganization in upper limp amputees. *Nature* 375, 482-484.

Flor, H., Mühlnickel, W., Karl, A., Denke, C., Grüsser, S., Taub, E., 2000. A neural substrate for nonpainful phantom-limb phenomena. *NeuroReport* 11, 1-5.

Flor, H., Denke, C., Schaefer, M., Grüsser, S., 2001. Effect of sensory discrimination on cortical reorganisation and phantom-limb pain. *Lancet* 357, 1763-1764.

Franz, E.A., Zelaznik, H.N., McCabe, G., 1991. Spatial topologixal constraints in a bimanual task. *Acta Psychol.* 77, 137-151.

Franz, E.A., 1997. Spatial coupling in the coordination of complex actions. *Q. J. Exp. Psychol.* 50, 684-704.

Franzen, J., 2001. The corrections. New York, Picador.

Gazzaniga, M., 1970. The bisected brain. New York: Appleton-Century-Crofts.

Gallese, V., Fadiga, L., Fogassi, L., Rizolatti , G., 1996. Action recognition in the premotor cortex. *Brain* 119, 593-609.

Gangitano, M., Mottaghy, F.M., Pascual-Leone, A., 2001. Phase-specific modulation of cortical motor output during movement observation. *Neuroreport* 12, 1489-1492.

Goldstein, K., 1908. Zur Lehre von der motorischen Apraxie. *J. Psychol. Neurol.* 11, 169-187.

Goodwin, G.M., McCloskey, D.I., Mathews, P.B.C., 1972. The contribution of muscle afferents to kinaesthesia shown by vibration induced illusions of movement and by the effects of paralysing joint afferents. *Brain* 95, 705-748.

Grafton, S.T., Arbib, M.A., Fadiga, L., Rizzolatti, G., 1996. Localization of grasp representations in humans by PET. 2. Observation compared with imagination. *Exp. Brain Res.* 112, 103-111.

Graziano, M.S., Yap, G.S., Gross, C.G., 1994. Coding of visual space by premotor neurons. *Science* 266, 1054-1057.

Graziano, M.S., 1999. Where is my arm? The relative role of vision and proprioception in the neuronal representation of limb position. *Prod. Natl. Acad. Sci. USA* 96, 1021-1034.

Graziano, M.S.A., Cooke, D.F., Taylor, C.S.R., 2000. Coding the location of the arm by sight. *Science* 290, 1782-1786.

Grüsser, S.M., Mühlnickel, W., Schaefer, M., Villringer, K., Christmann, C., Koeppe, C., Flor, H., 2004. Remote activation of referred phantom sensation and cortical reorganization in human upper extremity amputees. *Exp. Brain Res.* 154, 97-102.

Guillery, R.W., Feig, S.L., Lozsádi, D.A., 1998. Paying attention to the thalamic reticular nucleus *Trends Neurosci.* 21, 28-32.

Hägni, K., Eng, K., Hepp-Raymond, M.-C., Holper, L., Keisker, B., Siekierka, E., Kiper, D.C., 2008. Observing virtual arms that you imagine are yours increases the galvanic skin response to an unexpected threat. *PloS One* 3, e3082.

Hari, R., Karhu, J., Hämläinen, M., Knuutila, J., Salonen, O., Sams, M., Vilkman, V., 1993. Functional organization of the human first and second somatosensory cortices. A neuromagnetic study. *J. Neurosci.* 5, 724-734.

Hari, R., Hänninen, R., Mäkinen, T., Jousmäki, V., Forss, N., Seppä, M., Salonen, O., 1998. Three hands: fragmentation of human bodily awareness. *Neurosci. Lett.* 240, 131-134.

Harris, A.J., 1999. Cortical origin of pathological pain. *Lancet* 354, 1464-1467.

Head, H., Holmes, G., 1911. Sensory disturbances from cerebral lesions. *Brain* 34, 102-254.

Heidegger, M., 1927. Sein und Zeit, Max Niemeyer Verlag, Tübingen [German].

Hunter, J.P., Katz, J., Davis, K.D., 2003. The effect of tactile and visual sensory inputs on phantom-limb awareness. *Brain* 126, 579-589.

Iriki, A, Tanaka, M, Iwamura, Y., 1996. Coding a modified body schema during tool use by macaque postcentral neurones. *Neuroreport* 7, 2325-2330.

Iacoboni, M., Woods, R.P., Brass, M., Bekkering, H., Mazziotta, J.C., Rizzolatti, G., 1999. Cortical mechanisms of human imitation. *Science* 286, 2526-2528.

Iacoboni, M., Molnar-Szakacs, I., Gallese, V., Buccino, G., Mazziotta, J.C., Rizzolatti, G., 2005. Grasping the intentions of others with one's own mirror neuron system. *PLoS Biology* 3, 529-535.

Iacoboni, M., Dapretto, M., 2006. The mirror neuron system and the consequences of its dysfunction. *Nature Rev. Neurosci.* 7, 942-951.

Inoue, K., Kawashima, R., Sugiura, M., Ogawa, A., Schormann, T., Zilles, K., Fukuda, H., 2001. Activation in the ipsilateral posterior parietal cortex during tool use: a pet study. *Neuroimage* 14, 1469-1475.

Iwamura, Y., 1998. Hierarchical somatosensory processing. *Curr. Opin. Neurobiol.* 8, 522-528.

Jensen, T.S., Krebs, B., Nielsen, J., et al., 1983. Phantom limb, phantom pain and stump pain in amputees during the first 6 months following limb amputation. *Pain* 17, 243-56.

Kaas, J.H., Nelson, R.J., Sur, M., Lin, C.S., Merzenich, M.M., 1979. Multiple representations of the body within the primary somatosensory cortex of primates. *Science* 204, 521-523

Karl, A., Birbaumer, N., Lutzenberger, W., Cohen, L., Flor, H., 2001. Reorganization of motor and somatosensory cortex in upper extremity amputation with phantom-limb pain. *J. Neurosci.* 15, 3609-3618.

Keysers, C., Wicker, B., Gazzola, V., Anton, J.-L., Fogassi, L., Gallese, V., 2004. A touching sight: SII/PV activation during the observation and experience of touch. *Neuron* 42, 335-346.

Kennett, S., Taylor-Clarke, M., Haggard, P., 2001. Noninformative vision improves the spatial resolution of touch in humans. *Curr. Biol.* 11, 1188-1191.

Knight, R.T., Staines, W.R., Swick, D., Chao, L.L., 1999. Prefrontal cortex *Acta Psychol.* 101, 159-178.

Lackner, J.R., 1988. Some proprioceptive influences on the perceptual representation of body shape and orientation. *Brain* 111, 281-297.

Lenggenhager, B., Tadi, T., Metzinger, T., Blanke, O., 2007. Video ergo sum: manipulating bodily self-consciousness. *Science* 317, 1096-1099.

Makin, T.R., Holmes, N.P., Ehrsson, H.H., 2008. On the other hand: Dummy hands and peripersonal Space. *Behav. Brain Res.* 191, 1-10.

McAlonan, K., Brown, V.J., Bowman, E.M., 2000. Thalamic reticular nucleus activation reflects attentional gating during classical conditioning. *J. Neurosci.* 20, 8897-8901.

McGonigle, D.J., Hänninen, R., Salenius, S., Hari, R., Frackowiak, R.S., Frith, C.D., 2002. Whose arm is it anyway? An fMRI case study of supernumerary phantom limb. *Brain* 125, 1265-1274.

Merleau-Ponty, M., 1945. Phénoménologie de la perception. Paris, Gallimard.

Merzenich, M.M., Nelson, R.J., Stryker, M.P., Cynader, M.S., Schoppmann, A., Zook, J.M., 1984. Somatosensory cortical map changes following digit amputation in adult monkeys. *J. Comp. Neurol.* 224, 591-605.

Mitchell, S.W., 1871. Phantom limbs. *Lippincott's Magazine* 8, 563-569.

Mitchell, S.W., 1872. Injuries of nerves, and their consequences. Philadelphia, J.B. Lippincott.

Mountcastle, V.B., Powell, T.P., 1959. Central nervous mechanisms subserving position sense and kinesthesis. *Bull. Johns Hopkins Hosp.* 105, 173-200.

Moore, C.I., Nelson, S.B., 1998. Spatio-temporal subthreshold receptive fields in the vibrissa representation of rat primary somatosensory cortex. *J. Neurophysiol.* 80, 2882-2892.

Mühlnickel, W., Elbert, T., Taub, E., Flor, H., 1998. Reorganization of auditory cortex in tinnitus. *Proc Natl Acad Aci USA* 95, 10340-10343.

Newport, R., Hindle, J.V., Jackson, S.R., 2001. Links between vision and somatosensation. Vision can improve the felt position of the unseen hand. *Curr. Biol.* 11, 975-980.

Noppeney, U., Waberski, T.D., Gobbelé, R., Buchner, H., 1999. Spatial attention modulates the cortical somatosensory representation of the digits in humans. *NeuroReport* 10, 3137-3141.

Nicolelis, M.A., Fanselow, E.E., 2002. Thalamocortical optimization of tactile processing according to behavioral state. *Nat. Neurosci.* 5, 517-523.

Obayashi, S., Suhara, T., Kawabe, K., Okauchi, T., Maeda, J., Akine, Y., Hirotaka, O., Iriki, A., 2001. Functional brain mapping of monkey tool use. *Neuroimage* 14, 853-861.

Pavani, F., Spence, C., Driver, J., 2000. Visual capture of touch: Out-of-the-body experiences with rubber gloves. *Psychol. Sci.* 11, 353-359.

Peled, A., Pressman, A., Geva, A.B., Modai, I., 2003. Somatosensory evoked potentials during a rubber-hand illusion in schizophrenia. *Schizoph. Res.* 64, 157-163.

Penfield, W., Boldrey, E., 1937. Somatic motor and sensory representation in cerebral cortex of man as studied by electrical stimulation. *Brain* 60, 389-443.

Pavani, F., Spence, C., Driver, J., 2000. Visual capture of touch: Out-of-the-body experiences with rubber gloves. *Psychol. Sci.* 11, 353-359.

Petkova, A., Ehrsson, H.H., 2008. If I were you: perceptual illusion of body swapping. *PLOS One* 3, e3832.

Petkova, A., Ehrsson, HH., 2009. When right feels left: referral of touch and ownership between the hands. *PLOS One* 4, e6933.

Pleger, B., Dinse, H.R., Ragert, P., Schwenkreis, P., Malin, J.P., Tegenthoff, M., 2001. Shifts in cortical representations predict human discrimination improvement. *Proc. Natl. Acad. Sci.* 98, 12255-12260.

Pons, T., Garraghty, P.E., Ommaya, A., Kaas, J.H., Taub, E., Mishkin, M., 1991. Massive cortical reorganization after sensory deafferentation in adult macaques. *Science* 252, 1857-1860.

Ramachandran, V.S., Rogers-Ramachandran, D., 1996. Synaesthesia in phantom limbs induced with mirrors. *Proc. R. Soc. Lond. B Biol. Sci.* 263, 377-386.

Ramachandran, V.S., 1998. Consciousness and body image, lessons from phantom limbs, Capgras syndrome and pain asymbolia. *Phil. Trans. R. Soc. Lond. B* 353, 1851-1859.

Ramachandran, V.S., Hirstein, W., 1998. The perception of phantom limbs: The D.O. Hebb lecture. *Brain* 121, 1603-1630.

Riddoch, G., 1941. Phantom limbs and body shape. *Brain* 64, 197-222.

Rizzolatti, G., Fogassi, L., Gallese, V., 2001. Neurophysiological mechanisms underlying the understanding and imitation of action. *Nat. Rev. Neurosci.* 2, 661-670.

Rock, I., Victor, J., 1964. Vision and touch: An experimentally created conflict between the two senses. *Science* 143, 594-596.

Rockland, K.S., Ojima, H., 2003. Multisensory convergence in calcarine viusal areas in macaque monkey. *Intern. J. Psychophysiol.* 50, 19-26.

Rizzolatti, G., Fadiga, L., Gallese, V, Fogassi, L., 1996a. Premotor cortex and the recognition of motor actions. *Cog. Brain Res.* 3, 131-141.

Rizzolatti, G., Fadiga, L., Matelli, M., Bettinardi, V., Paulesu, E., Perani, D., Fazio, F., 1996b. Localization of grasp representations in humans by PET. *Exp. Brain Res.* 111, 246-252.

Rizzolatti, G., Fogassi, L. Gallese, V., 2001. Neurophysiological mechanisms underlying the understanding and imitation of action. *Nat. Neurosci.* 2, 661-670.

Ro, T., Wallace, R., Hagedorn, J., Farne, A., Pienkos, E., 2004. Visual enhancing of tactile perception in the posterior parietal cortex. *J. Cogn. Neurosci.* 16, 24-30.

Rockland, K.S., Ojima, H., 2003. Multisensory convergence in calcarine viusal areas in macaque monkey. *Intern. J. Psychophysiol.* 50, 19-26.

Rorden, C., Heutink, J., Greenfield, E., Robertson, I.H., 1999. When a rubber hand "feels" what the real hand cannot. *NeuroReport* 10, 135-138.

Sadato, N., Yonekura, Y., Waki, A., Yamada, H., Ishii, Y., 1997. Role of the supplementary motor area and the right premotor cortex in the coordination of bimanual finger movements. *J. Neurosci.* 17, 9667-9674.

Sathian, K., Greenspan, A.I., Wolf, S.L. 2000. Doing it with mirrors: a case study of a novel approach to neurorehabilitation. *Neurorehabil. Neural. Repair* 14, 73-76.

Schaefer, M., Mühlnickel, W., Grüsser, S.M., Flor, H., 2002. Reproducibility and stability of neuroelectric source imaging in primary somatosensory cortex. *Brain Topogr.* 14, 179-189.

Schaefer, M., Mühlnickel, W., Grüsser, S.M., Flor, H., 2002. Reliability and validity of neuroelectric source imaging in primary somatosensory cortex of human upper limb amputees. *Brain Topogr.* 15, 95-106.

Schaefer, M., Noennig, N., Karl, A., Heinze, H.-J., Rotte, M., 2004a. Reproducibility and stability of neuromagnetic source imaging in primary somatosensory cortex. *Brain Topogr.* 17, 47-53.

Schaefer, M., Rothemund, Y., Heinze, H.-J., Rotte, M., 2004b. Short-time plasticity of the primary somatosensory cortex during tool use: a MEG study. *NeuroReport* 15, 1293-1297.

Schaefer, M., Flor, H., Heinze, H.-J., Rotte M., 2005a. Dynamic shifts in the organization of primary somatosensory cortex induced by bimanual spatial coupling of motor activity. *Neuroimage* 25, 395-400.

Schaefer, M., Heinze, H.-J., Rotte, M., 2005b. Task-relevant modulation of primary somatosensory cortex suggests a prefrontal-cortical sensory gating system. *Neuroimage* 17, 130-135.

Schaefer, M., Heinze, H.-J., Rotte, M., 2005c. Seeing the hand being touched modulates the primary somatosensory cortex. *NeuroReport* 13, 1101-1115.

Schaefer, M., Noennig, N., Heinze, H.-J., Rotte, M., 2006a. Fooling your feelings: Artificially induced referred sensations are linked to a modulation of the primary somatosensory cortex. *Neuroimage* 29, 67-73.

Schaefer, M., Flor, H., Heinze, H.-J., Rotte, M., 2006b. Dynamic modulation of the primary somatosensory cortex during seeing and feeling a touched hand. *Neuroimage* 29, 587-592.

Schaefer, M., Flor, H., Heinze, H.-J., Rotte, M., 2007. Morphing the body: illusory feeling of an elongated arm affects somatosensory homunculus. *Neuroimage* 36, 700-705.

Schaefer, M., Heinze, H.-J., Rotte, M., 2008a. Seeing the hand bigger than it is: Observing the touched body magnified alters somatosensory homunculus. *NeuroReport* 19, 901-905.

Schaefer, M., Heinze, H.-J., Rotte, M., 2008b. My third arm: feeling an artificial supernumerary arm changes topography of the homunculus. Human Brain Mapping, in press.

Schaefer, M., Xu, B., Flor, H., Cohen, L.G., 2009. Effects of different viewing perspectives on somatosensory activations during observation of touch. Human Brain Mapping, in press.

Sadato, N., Yonekura, Y., Waki, A., Yamada, H., Ishii, Y., 1997. Role of the supplementary motor area and the right premotor cortex in the coordination of bimanuall finger movements. *J. Neurosci.* 17, 9667-9674.

Sellal, F., Renaseau-Leclerc, C., Labrecque, R., 1996. The man with 6 arms. An analysis of supernumerary phantom limbs after right hemisphere stroke. *Rev. Neurol. (Paris)* 152, 190-195 [French].

Serino, A., Farnè, A., Rinaldesi, M.L., Haggard, P., Làdavas, E., 2007. Can vision of the body ameliorate impaired somatosensory function? *Neuropsychologia* 45, 1101-1107.

Serino, A., Haggard, P., 2009. Touch and the body. *Neurosci. Biobehav. Rev.*, in press.

Shallice, T., 1982. Specific impairments of planning. *Philos. Trans. R. Soc. Lond. B Biol. Sci.* 98, 199-209.

Shmuclof, L., Zohary, E. 2008. Mirror-image representation of action in the anterior parietal cortex. *Nat. Neursoci.* 11, 1267-1269.

Simon, H.A., 1975. The functional equivalence of problem-solving skill. *Cogn. Psychol.* 7, 268-288.

Skinner, J.E., Yingling, C.D., 1976. Regulation of slow potential shifts in nucleus reticularis thalami by the mesencephalic reticular formation and the frontal granular cortex. Electroencephalogr. *Clin. Neurophysiol.* 41, 476-482.

Staines, W.R., Graham, S.J., Black, S.E., McIlroy, W.E., 2002. Task-relevant modulation of contralateral and ipsilateral primary somatosensory cortex and the role of a prefrontal-cortical sensory gating system. *Neuroimage* 15, 190-199.

Stefan, K., Cohen, L.G., Duque, J., Mazzocchio, R., Celnik, P., Sawaki, L., Ungerleider, L., Classen, J., 2005. Formation of a motor memory by action observation. *J. Neurosci.* 25, 9339-9346.

Steyvers, M., Etoh, S., Sauner, D., Levin, O., Siebner, H.R., Swinnen, S.P., Rothwell, J.C., 2003. High-frequency transcranial magnetic stimulation of the supplementary motor area reduces bimanual coupling during anti-phase but not in-phase movements. *Exp. Brain Res.* 151, 309-317.

Taylor-Clarke, M., Kennett, S., Haggard, P., 2002. Vision modulates somatosensory cortical processing. *Curr. Biol.* 12, 233-236.

Taylor-Clarke, M., Jacobsen, P., Haggard, P., 2004. Keeping the world a constant size: object constancy in human touch. *Nat. Neurosci.* 7, 219-220.

Tastevin, J., 1937. En partant de l'experience d'Aristotele. *L'Encephale* 1, 57-84.

Wartan, S.W., Hamann, W., Wedley, J.R. , McColl, I., 1997. Phantom pain and sensation among British veteran amputees. *British J. Anaesth.* 78, 652-659.

Weinstein, E.A., Kahn, R.L., Malitz, S., Rozanski, J., 1954. Delusional reduplication of parts of the body. *Brain* 77, 45-60.

Welch, R.B., 1972. The effect of experienced limb identity upon adaptation to simulated displacement of the visual field. *Percept. Psychophys.* 12, 453-456.

Wheeler, M.E., Petersen, S.E., Buckner, R.I., 2000. Memory's echo: vivid remembering reactivates sensory-specific cortex. *Proc. Natl. Acad. Aci. USA* 97, 11125-11129.

Yang, T.T., Gallen, C., Schwartz, B., Bloom, F.E., Ramachandran, V.S., Cobb, S., 1994. Sensory maps in the human brain. *Nature* 36, 592-593.

Yamaguchi, S., Knight, R.T., 1990. Gating of somatosensory input by human prefrontal cortex. *Brain Res.* 531, 281-288.

Yamamoto, S., Kitazawa, S., 2001. Sensation at the tips of invisible tools. *Nat. Neurosci.* 4, 979-980.

Zhou, Y.D., Fuster, J.M., 1997. Neuronal activity of somatosensory cortex in a cross-modal (visuo-haptic) memory task. *Exp. Brain Res.* 116, 551-555.

Zhou, Y.D., Fuster, J.M., 2000. Visuo-tactile cross-modal associations in cortical somatosensory cells. *Proc. Natl. Acad. Sci. USA* 97, 9777-9782.

Zhu, Z., Nagarajan, S.S., Zumer, J.M., McGonigle, D.J., Disbrow, E.A., 2007. Spatiotemporal integration of tactile information in human somatosensory cortex. *BMC Neurosci.* 14, 21.

INDEX

A

activation, 17, 19, 23, 24, 26, 42, 50, 51, 52, 53, 54, 56, 58, 71, 74, 75, 76
adults, 2, 6
agent, 53, 56
amputation, 3, 5, 6, 7, 23, 24, 49, 62, 75, 76
anorexia, 42, 66
anorexia nervosa, 42, 66
ANOVA, 16, 31
appetite, 35
argument, 62, 68
artery, 56
assessment, 50, 54
assimilation, 11
attribution, 2, 53
auditory cortex, 66, 76
awareness, 74, 75

B

bad day, 55
basal ganglia, 12, 42, 56
behavior, 3, 49, 50, 56, 57, 58
beneficial effect, 61, 63
bleeding, 43
blocks, 13
blood, 67
body image, ix, 2, 6, 8, 11, 12, 16, 39, 41, 42, 43, 44, 46, 58, 66, 77
body schema, 12, 13, 16, 45, 75
body shape, 38, 75, 77
body size, 39, 40
brain, 1, 2, 6, 8, 12, 13, 14, 24, 26, 30, 39, 42, 44, 45, 46, 48, 50, 52, 53, 54, 56, 57, 58, 59, 61, 62, 63, 65, 66, 67, 69, 73, 76
brain activity, 13, 24, 58

C

case study, 3, 33, 42, 56, 76, 78
cell, 11
cerebellum, 12
cerebral cortex, 76
childhood, 6
classical conditioning, 76
clinical trials, 62, 63
coding, 66
cognition, 19, 42
cognitive function, 46
cognitive variables, 42, 66
components, 31
conflict, 25, 26, 43, 58, 59, 73, 77
connectivity, 52
consciousness, 68
contralateral hemisphere, 12, 54
control, 9, 12, 13, 19, 20, 24, 28, 31, 37, 38, 40, 41, 50, 55, 56, 57, 60, 61, 63, 67, 69
control condition, 12, 13, 24, 28, 31, 37, 38, 40, 41, 50, 61

control group, 9, 57, 60, 67
convergence, 72, 77, 78
corpus callosum, 56
correlation, 17, 67
cortex, ix, 2, 6, 7, 12, 15, 16, 17, 19, 23, 26, 27, 30, 34, 39, 40, 42, 46, 50, 52, 54, 56, 57, 58, 66, 67, 71, 72, 73, 75, 76, 77, 78, 79, 80
corticobasal degeneration, 56, 57
coupling, 17, 73, 78, 80
covering, 9

D

death, 5
decisions, 68
depression, 2
destruction, 5
detection, 58
diaphragm, 13, 14, 28
differentiation, 53, 67
discrimination, 9, 28, 31, 61, 71, 73, 77
discrimination tasks, 61, 71
discrimination training, 9
discs, 19
disorder, 3, 55, 56
displacement, 17, 18, 80
dissociation, 53
distortions, 8, 36, 43, 44, 59, 66
distress, 42
dominance, 25, 40, 43, 44
dorsolateral prefrontal cortex, 26
dream, 35
duplication, 49
duration, 9
dystonia, 26

E

eating, 69
EEG, 9, 28
ego, 54
electroencephalography, 9
emotions, 69
enlargement, 25, 38
enthusiasm, 62
environment, 1, 2, 13
evoked potential, 46, 76
execution, 17, 49
experimental condition, 25, 31, 50

F

feedback, 9, 18, 26, 30, 39, 42, 43, 62, 66
feelings, 2, 5, 35, 36, 42, 46, 78
flexibility, 69
focusing, ix
food, 11, 35, 69
frontal lobe, 3, 16, 56

G

genre, 6
grants, 69
groups, 43

H

hallucinations, 67, 72
hands, 2, 13, 17, 30, 31, 43, 45, 46, 48, 49, 51, 54, 55, 56, 58, 59, 61, 62, 68, 72, 74, 75, 77
handwriting, 17
height, 13, 35
hemiparesis, 62, 71
hemisphere, 31
human brain, 80
human subjects, ix, 12, 24
hypothesis, 3, 13, 17, 23, 24, 28, 37, 40, 59

I

identity, 2, 80
illusion, ix, 23, 24, 25, 26, 36, 37, 38, 39, 40, 41, 42, 43, 46, 47, 48, 57, 58, 59, 62, 71, 72, 76, 77
illusions, ix, 3, 24, 25, 36, 41, 42, 46, 48, 59, 65, 74
imagery, 43, 67
images, 1, 14, 36, 66

imagination, 53, 74
imitation, 53, 75, 77
impairments, 34, 79
indirect effect, 38
induction, 57, 73
infection, 56
inferences, 49
injuries, 8
integration, ix, 9, 12, 24, 26, 36, 46, 59, 61, 63, 80
intentionality, 53, 68
intentions, 53, 68, 75
interaction, 2, 27, 31, 50, 62
interaction effect, 31
interactions, 27, 30, 50
interdependence, 27
ipsilateral, 12, 19, 31, 75, 79

J

joints, 17

K

kinesthesis, 76

L

learning, 9
left hemisphere, 15
lesions, 42, 56, 57, 74
light beam, 46
links, 27
localization, 14, 18, 28

M

magnetic field, 14, 16
magnetoencephalography, 8
mammalian brain, 6
manipulation, 26, 39, 43, 46, 57, 58, 66
mapping, 13, 49, 76
Martin Heidegger, 68
median, 9
MEG, 8, 13, 14, 24, 25, 28, 47, 67, 78
memory, 33, 72, 79, 80
Merleau-Ponty, 6, 68, 76
metamorphosis, 35, 36
metaphor, 35
modeling, 14
morning, 35, 55
motion, 16, 31, 32, 50
motor actions, 17, 77
motor activity, 16, 71, 78
motor system, 26
motor task, 17, 19, 21, 34
movement, 3, 17, 33, 55, 56, 57, 62, 74
MRI, 15, 18, 20, 38
muscles, 17

N

nausea, 26
nerve, 9
network, 39, 56, 65, 66
neural connection, 6
neural network, 13, 16, 53, 56
neural systems, 56
neurodegenerative disorders, 57
neuroimaging, 3, 6, 58
neurological disease, 56
neurons, 11, 17, 21, 26, 27, 33, 34, 39, 49, 50, 74
neuroscience, 65, 68
nucleus, 21, 74, 76, 79

O

observations, 65
occipital lobe, 2
openness, 68
optimization, 76
orientation, 75
ownership, 2, 46, 49, 57, 58, 73, 77
oxygen, 67

P

pain, 3, 5, 6, 7, 8, 9, 12, 26, 44, 61, 62, 63, 66, 73, 74, 75, 77, 80
paralysis, 62
parietal cortex, 11, 12, 40, 46, 50, 52, 54, 58, 75, 77, 79
parietal lobe, 26, 56, 57
passive, 58
perceptions, 66
PET, 12, 74, 77
phalanges, 28
philosophers, 1, 6, 55, 68
physical therapy, 9
physics, 65
physiology, 68
planning, 19, 57, 79
plasticity, 6, 9, 78
positron, 12
positron emission tomography, 12
prefrontal cortex, 19, 80
problem-solving, 19, 79
problem-solving behavior, 19
prototype, 19
pulse, 13, 14, 28

R

range, 1, 61
ratings, 67
reality, 62, 66
reasoning, 2
receptive field, 12, 39, 52, 76
receptors, 44
recognition, 49, 50, 53, 73, 77
recovery, 6, 51
reflection, 23, 39, 62
regulations, 19
rehabilitation, 51, 62, 66
relationship, 1, 65
remote sensing, 44
René Descartes, 68
reproduction, 1
resolution, 75
responsiveness, 21
right hemisphere, 15, 79
rings, 19, 58
rubber, 13, 33, 36, 42, 43, 46, 47, 48, 57, 58, 59, 61, 73, 76, 77, 78

S

sample, 60, 63
schema, 11, 12, 16
schizophrenia, 76
schizophrenic patients, 46, 57, 67
selecting, 19
self-consciousness, 75
sensation, 5, 11, 13, 14, 23, 24, 25, 26, 28, 40, 74, 80
sensations, 7, 12, 13, 24, 26, 44, 46, 49, 62, 66, 71, 78
sensitivity, 6, 31, 32, 33, 54, 61
sensors, 14, 15
shape, 2, 11, 17, 24, 36, 39, 40, 43
short-term memory, 50
signals, 13, 59
signs, 56
SII, 12, 13, 16, 26, 51, 53, 71, 75
simulation, 54, 72
skills, 63
skin, ix, 2, 13, 14, 17, 23, 24, 27, 28, 43, 61, 66, 71, 74
social context, 54
social perception, ix, 46, 65
social situations, 53
somatosensory function, 33, 34, 79
Spain, 5
speech, 67
stability, 61, 78
stages, 24, 36, 42, 66, 67, 68
stimulus, 15, 16, 20, 21, 23, 27, 33, 50
strategies, 51
strength, 40, 42, 55, 58
stroke, 3, 33, 51, 61, 62, 71, 72, 79
suppression, 19
switching, 21
symptom, 56
syndrome, 3, 55, 56, 57, 59, 71, 77

T

tactile stimuli, 7, 13, 24, 27, 30
task demands, 17, 21
tendon, 39
thalamus, 26
therapeutic approaches, 9, 44, 61
therapy, 62, 63
thinking, 2
threat, 74
threshold, 21, 31, 32
thresholds, 31
tinnitus, 66, 76
tradition, 35, 68
traditional views, 25, 45, 66, 67
training, 9, 16, 33, 51, 61, 62, 63, 72
trajectory, 17
transformations, 35

V

validity, 63, 78
variance, 14
vibration, 74
vision, 24, 26, 27, 30, 33, 42, 43, 44, 50, 59, 62, 66, 71, 74, 75, 76, 79
visual field, 80
visual modality, 25, 40, 43
visual stimuli, 27, 31, 32, 33, 50
visual stimulus, 28, 50

W

waking, 35
war, 7
wear, 36, 40
West Africa, 5
wood, 19